PEDIATRIC DERMATOLOGY AND DERMATOPATHOLOGY

PEDIATRIC DERMATOLOGY AND DERMATOPATHOLOGY

A CONCISE ATLAS

Ruggero Caputo MD

Professor and Chairman
Istituto di Scienze Dermatologiche
Università di Milano
IRCCS Ospedale Maggiore
Milan, Italy

Carlo Gelmetti MD

Associated Professor
Istituto di Scienze Dermatologiche
Università di Milano
IRCCS Ospedale Maggiore
Milan, Italy

MARTIN DUNITZ

© 2002, Martin Dunitz Ltd, a member of the Taylor & Francis group

First published in the United Kingdom in 2002 by
Martin Dunitz Ltd
The Livery House
7–9 Pratt Street
London NW1 0AE

Tel: +44-(0)20-7482-2202
Fax: +44-(0)20-7267-0159
E-mail: info@dunitz.co.uk
Website: http://www.dunitz.co.uk

Although every effort is made to ensure that drug doses and other information are
presented accurately in this publication, the ultimate responsibility rests with the
prescribing physician. Neither the publishers nor the authors can be held responsible
for errors or for any consequences arising from the use of information contained
herein.

A CIP catalogue record for this book is available from the British Library

ISBN 1-84184-120-X

Distributed in the USA by
Fulfilment Center
Taylor & Francis
7625 Empire Drive
Florence, KY 41042, USA
Toll Free Tel: 1-800-634-7064
Email: cserve@routledge_ny.com

Distributed in Canada by
Taylor & Francis
74 Rolark Drive
Scarborough
Ontario M1R 4G2, Canada
Toll Free Tel: 1-877-226-2237
Email: tal_fran@istar.ca

Distributed in the rest of the world by
ITPS Limited
Cheriton House
North Way, Andover
Hampshire SP10 5BE, UK
Tel: +44-(0)1264 332424
Email: reception@itps.co.uk

Composition by Scribe Design, Gillingham, Kent, UK
Front cover image: Angel Playing the Lute, 1515 (panel) by Giovanni Battista di Jacopo
'Rosso Fiorentino' (1494–1540), Galleria degli Uffizi, Florence, Italy/Bridgeman Art Library.
Printed and bound in Singapore by Kyodo

CONTENTS

PREFACE

It is almost ten years since the first volume of *Pediatric Dermatology and Dermatopathology* was published. The original, four-volume textbook represents the synthesis of the clinical experience of the Milan school of pediatric dermatology and the unrivalled expertise of US dermatopathologists. This landmark text built on the tradition of the late Professor Ferdinando Giannotti; and Bernard Akerman and his co-workers, among whom we would like to mention Evita Sison-Torre and Giorgio Annessi, made an invaluable contribution providing all the histological images.

At present, pediatric dermatology is a fast-growing specialty, and there is a real need for educational resources. It is with this in mind that we have decided to bring together a concise edition of *Pediatric Dermatology and Dermatopathology* in one single, accessible volume. The text has been revised to take account of the latest developments in the field, some of the old chapters have been deleted and new ones have been added. The illustrations have been selected to offer a comprehensive distillation of the original textbook.

Ruggero Caputo
Carlo Gelmetti

ACKNOWLEDGEMENTS

We would like to thank Gianluca Tadini for revising the chapters on genodermatosis. In particular, our thanks go to Bernard Ackerman for his generosity in allowing us to use his unique collection of histological images. We also wish to thank Dr R. Gianotti for the new histological slides, Professor G.H. Findlay and Dr L. Smith, who provided clinical photographs of black children, and Professor Y.K. Zhao, who contributed all the pictures of Asian children.

ACANTHOSIS NIGRICANS

Acanthosis nigricans manifests itself as dark, soft plaques with papillated surfaces. It has a predilection for the flexures. It may develop *de novo* or in response to a variety of systemic disorders.

EPIDEMIOLOGY

Acanthosis nigricans is rare in children and usually develops after infancy.

CLINICAL FINDINGS

The earliest change – tan, dark brown or black pigmentation with accentuation of skin markings – typically affects the axillae, the back and sides of the neck (Fig. 1.1), the groin (Fig. 1.2), the perineum and the antecubital fossae. The plaques may be studded by acrochordon-like excrescencies of different sizes. Acanthosis nigricans involves the oral cavity in nearly half of the patients; more rarely it involves the anogenital mucosa (see Fig. 1.2).

LABORATORY FINDINGS

Children with acanthosis nigricans may have overt diabetes.

HISTOPATHOLOGICAL FINDINGS

All forms of acanthosis nigricans are characterized by marked papillomatosis (see Figs 1.3 and 1.4) (i.e. dermal papillae that project above the surface of the contiguous normal skin). The epidermis is thinned rather than acanthotic, and it is usually only slightly hyperpigmented.

ETIOLOGY AND PATHOGENESIS

Acanthosis nigricans is probably caused by activation of receptors for specific growth factors (e.g. insulin-like growth factors, epidermal growth factors) on the surface of keratinocytes. The traditional subdivision of acanthosis nigricans into a 'benign' form (not associated with any other disorder and occasionally familial), a 'malignant' form (paraneoplastic acanthosis nigricans), a 'syndromal' form (associated with endocrine disorders), a 'pseudo' form (in obese people) and a 'drug-induced' form is as incorrect pathophysiologially as it is morphologically. In fact, all forms of acanthosis nigricans have the same clinical and histopathological features.

COURSE

The course of acanthosis nigricans depends entirely on whether there is an underlying disease and, if there is, on its nature.

MANAGEMENT

The treatment is symptomatic. Underlying disorders should be treated as appropriate.

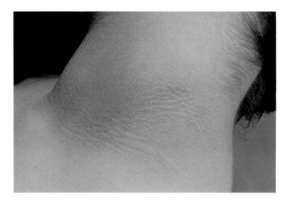

Figure 1.1
Acanthosis nigricans. Grey–brown papillated lesions situated between accentuation of normal skin creases on the neck.

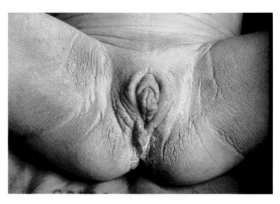

Figure 1.2
Acanthosis nigricans. Seip–Lawrence syndrome (generalized lipodystropy, diabetes mellitus, muscular hypertrophy, acromegaloid facies and early bone maturation). Prominent, brownish, confluent papillations accentuate the normal skin markings. The clitoris is hypertrophied.

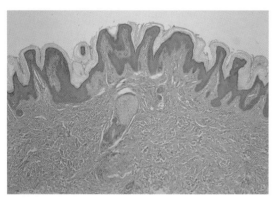

Figures 1.3 and 1.4
Acanthosis nigricans. Thin papillations are covered by cornified cells in a 'basket-weave' configuration. They are further characterized by thinned epidermis, thinned elongated dermal papillae and slight epidermal hyperpigmentation.

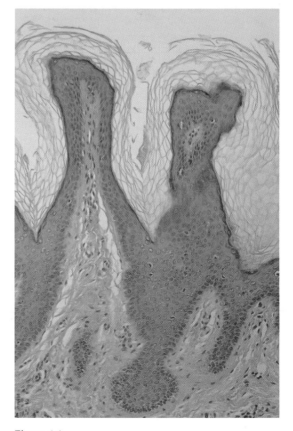

Figure 1.4

ACNEIFORM DISORDERS

Acne is an extremely common disorder of the folliculosebaceous unit. It may occur in the first year of life (acne neonatorum and acne infantum), but it is predominantly a disease of the second decade of life (acne vulgaris). Less frequent acneiform disorders are acne fulminans, drug-induced acne and chloracne.

ACNE VULGARIS

CLINICAL FINDINGS

The lesions of acne are polymorphic:

- comedones may be open ('blackheads') or closed ('whiteheads') (Fig. 2.1);
- papules with or without inflammation (Fig. 2.2);
- pustules caused by suppurative folliculitis (see Fig. 2.2, Fig. 2.3);
- nodules that develop after rupture of comedones or follicular cysts (see Fig. 2.3).

One type of lesion may predominate.
 The face, back, chest and shoulders are common sites.

COMPLICATIONS

Complications of acneiform disorders include:

- scars, which may be depressed or hypertrophic;
- excoriations induced by emotional factors;
- coalescence of nodules, cysts and abscesses with formation of interconnecting channels and sinus tracts (acne conglobata);

- post-inflammatory hyperpigmentation.

ETIOLOGY AND PATHOGENESIS

The clinical variety of lesions that typify acne result from an interplay of factors, such as:

- altered cornification of follicular infundibula;
- increased and altered secretion of sebum;
- proliferation of bacteria within infundubula;
- increased androgen activity.

COURSE

The course of acne is unpredictable. The lesions usually begin to decline at about the age of 20 years.

HISTOPATHOLOGICAL FINDINGS

Open comedones are follicular infundibula that have become widely dilated because of plugging with a markedly increased number of orthokeratotic cornified cells (Fig. 2.7).
 Closed comedones are tiny infundibular cysts that are filled with cornified cells, sebum and micro-organisms (Fig. 2.8).
 Pustules are collections of neutrophils that fill widened follicular infundibula.
 Inflammatory papules and nodules are suppurative granulomatous inflammation resulting from ruptured infundibular cysts (Fig. 2.9).

MANAGEMENT

Topical therapy

Topical treatments include:

- benzoyl peroxide (2.5%, 5% or 10%);
- retinoids (mainly for comedonic acne);
- antibiotics (clindamycin or erythromycin);
- azelaic acid.

Systemic therapy

Systemic treatments include:

- isotretinoin (0.5–1 mg/kg per day for 4–6 months for severe cases; 0.5 mg/kg per day for the first week of the month for 4–6 months for moderate cases);
- antibiotics (tetracycline, doxycycline, minocycline or erythromycin).

ACNE NEONATORUM AND ACNE INFANTUM

Acne neonatorum occurs before the third month of life.

The eruption of acne neonatorum and acne infantum is usually limited to a few comedones, papules or pustules, but in infants the lesions may be numerous (Fig. 2.4).The condition is believed to result from stimulation of fetal sebaceous glands by maternal hormones.

ACNE FULMINANS

Acne fulminans is seen exclusively in teenage boys. It is characterized by an explosive onset of large, reddish, exquisitely tender papules and nodules on the back and chest (Fig. 2.5). Ulceration ensues rapidly. The youth is febrile and complains of pain in the muscles or joints. Osteolytic lesions are sometimes present at sites of tenderness. Systemic corticosteroids and antibiotics must be initiated immediately if the process is to be brought under control.

DRUG-INDUCED ACNE

Topical and systemic corticosteroids, androgens, iodides, bromides, rifampicin (rifampin), isoniazid, phenobarbital, diphenylhydantoin and lithium carbonate have all been reported as causes of acneiform eruptions. The lesions in drug-induced acne consist of reddish papules and small pustules. Comedones and cystic nodules are rare.

CHLORACNE

Children exposed to dioxin for short periods develop only a few comedones, whereas those exposed for longer periods develop keratotic papules, large pustules, nodules and cysts, especially on the face (Fig. 2.6). Histopathologically, the lesions of chloracne show infundibula and eccrine ducts plugged by cornified cells and typical features of a suppurative folliculitis (Fig. 2.10).

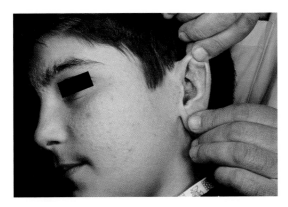

Figure 2.1
Acne vulgaris. There are numerous comedones on the ear, cheek, forehead and nose.

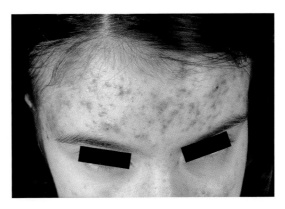

Figure 2.2

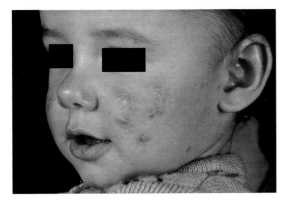

Figure 2.4
Acne infantum. Reddish papules and pustules coexist with atrophic scars.

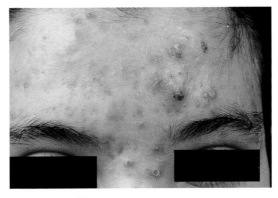

Figures 2.2 and 2.3
Acne vulgaris. The foreheads of the two girls are covered by typical lesions (comedones and pustules), on which are yellowish and hemorrhagic crusts.

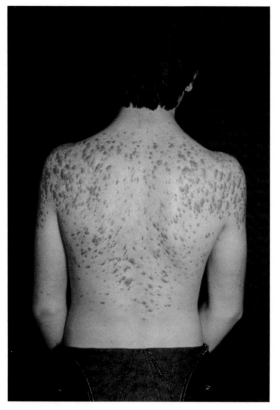

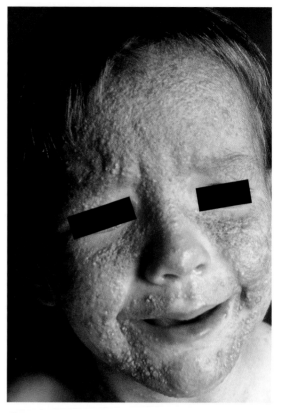

Figure 2.5
Acne fulminans. Widespread reddish papules and nodules are located in zones where sebaceous glands are most numerous. Each large lesion represents suppurative granulomatous inflammation in response to rupture of an infundibular cyst.

Figure 2.6
Chloracne. Diffuse involvement of comedones, papules and pustules, many of which are topped by crusts.

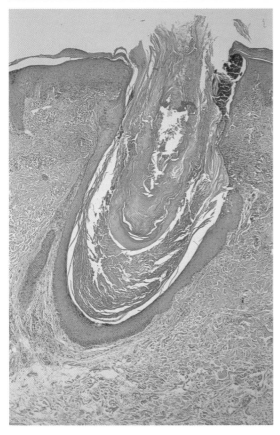

Figure 2.7
Acne vulgaris. Open comedones are simply follicular infundibula that have become widely dilated because of plugging by a markedly increased number of orthokeratotic cornified cells, which are arranged in laminated and compact fashion.

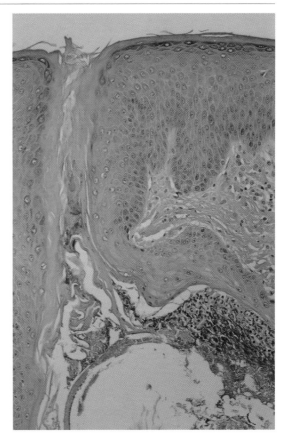

Fig. 2.9
Acne vulgaris showing suppurative folliculitis. There is an abscess within the dilated follicular infundibulum, with rupture of the infundibular epithelium.

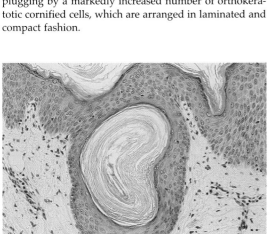

Figure 2.8
Acne vulgaris. Closed comedones are tiny infundibular cysts filled by cornified cells and sebum.

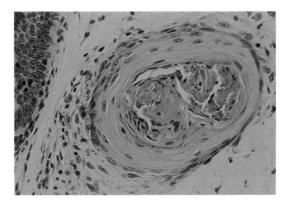

Figure 2.10
Chloracne. An eccrine dermal duct plugged by cornified cells.

3 ACQUIRED MELANOCYTIC NEVI

UNNA'S NEVI

CLINICAL FINDINGS

Unna's nevi are skin-colored or brown, soft, pedunculated or sessile lesions. They are sometimes papillomatous excrescences (Fig. 3.1). They often cannot be differentiated clinically from acrochordons. They are uncommon in children.

HISTOPATHOLOGICAL FINDINGS

Histology shows pedunculated or sessile lesion with nests, cords and strands of melanocytes within a markedly thickened exophytic papillary dermis. Some nests of melanocytes may be present at the dermoepidermal junction.

MIESCHER'S NEVI

CLINICAL FINDINGS

Miescher's nevi are globoid, smooth-surfaced, skin-colored or tan papules. They are almost always found on the face. Like Unna's nevi, they are uncommon in children.

HISTOPATHOLOGICAL FINDINGS

Histology shows dome-shaped nevi. They are usually intradermal but they may be compound. A wedge-shaped array of usually small, round melanocytes extend into the reticular dermis and occasionally into the subcutaneous fat (Fig. 3.2).

SPITZ'S NEVI

CLINICAL FINDINGS

Spitz's nevi are dome-shaped, smooth, firm, hairless, nodules. They are usually less than 10 mm in diameter. They are usually pink or red in color, but they may be tan, brown or even black. Spitz's nevi are usually solitary and favor the face, but they may occur anywhere on the integument (Figs 3.3 and 3.4). One-third of patients are aged under 10 years.

HISTOPATHOLOGICAL FINDINGS

Spitz's nevi are characterized by melanocytes with large nuclei and usually with abundant amphophilic cytoplasm and round, oval, polygonal or spindle shapes. Multinucleated or mononuclear giant melanocytes are commonly seen. Spitz's nevi evolve through junctional compound and intradermal stages. Junctional and compound types may show hyperkeratosis, hypergranulosis and the presence of dull, pink globules (Kamino bodies) within the epidermis (Figs 3.5 and 3.6).

CLARK'S NEVI

CLINICAL FINDINGS

Clark's nevi are often small, symmetrical, well-circumscribed macules or papules. They usually have a relatively uniform dark brownish color centrally with a lighter brown color peripherally. Occasionally they may be large (more than 10 mm in diameter), asymmetrical with scalloped or notched borders and variegated in shades of brown. Sites of predilection are the trunk and proximal part of extremities. Clark's nevi are the commonest type of acquired nevi (Fig. 3.7).

HISTOPATHOLOGICAL FINDINGS

Clark's nevi may be junctional, compound or intradermal. In junctional nevi, there are nests of melanocytes at the dermoepidermal junction. In compound nevi, nests of melanocytes at the dermoepidermal junction extend for some rete ridges beyond nests of melanocytes in the papillary dermis. In intradermal nevi, nests of melanocytes are in a thickened papillary dermis. Melanocytes tend to be small and oval and monomorphous (Fig. 3.8).

SUTTON'S NEVI

CLINICAL FINDINGS

Sutton's nevi (or halo nevi) are simply a distinctive variant of Clark's nevi around which a rim of depigmentation begins and extends centrifugally. The nevus is centrally located and eventually tends to disappear (in months or years) Sutton's nevi occur mainly on the trunk (Fig. 3.9).

HISTOPATHOLOGICAL FINDINGS

Histology shows a junctional or compound nevus surrounded by a lymphocytic infiltrate (Fig. 3.10).

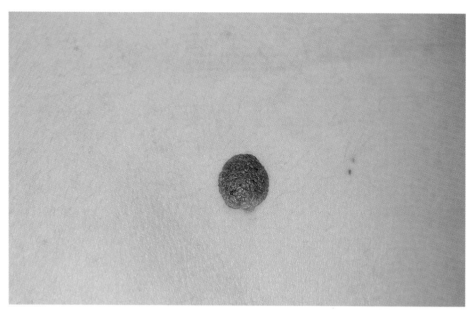

Figure 3.1
Unna's nevus. This papillomatous lesion is composed largely of nests, cords and strands of melanocytes in the dermis.

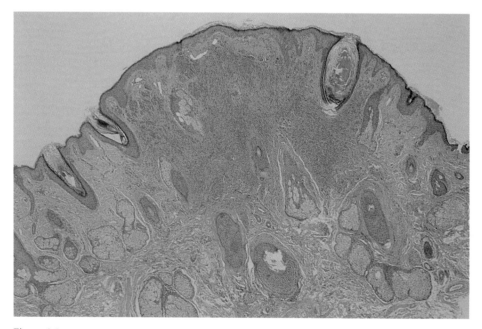

Figure 3.2
Miescher's nevus. This domed nevus is characterized by orderly nests, cords and strands of melanocytes that extend throughout the reticular dermis.

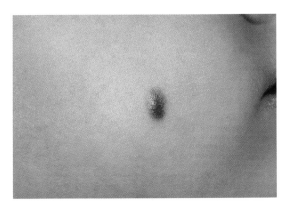

Figure 3.3
Spitz's nevus. The lesion is small, symmetrical, well circumscribed, smooth-surfaced and uniformly brown–red in color.

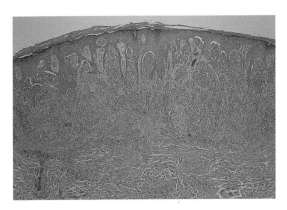

Figure 3.5

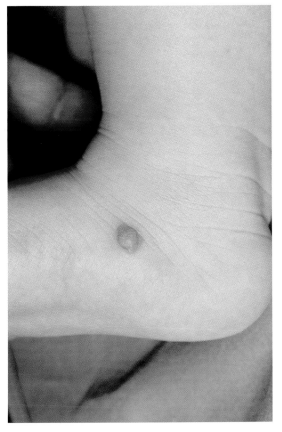

Figure 3.4
Spitz's nevus. The lesion is small, and the central dome-shaped portion is symmetrical. It is relatively well circumscribed, slightly scaly and pinkish red in color.

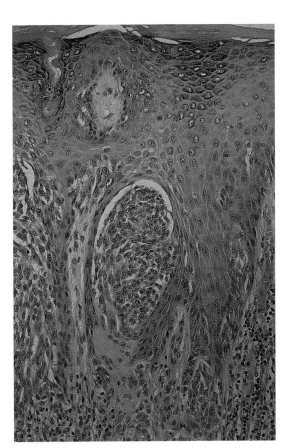

Figures 3.5 and 3.6
Spitz's nevus, compound type. In addition to epidermal and dermal oval-shaped melanocytes with relatively large nuclei, there is hyperkeratosis, hypergranulosis, irregular epidermal hyperplasia, clefts between elongated nests of melanocytes and surrounding keratinocytes, and dull pink globules (Kamino bodies) within the epidermis.

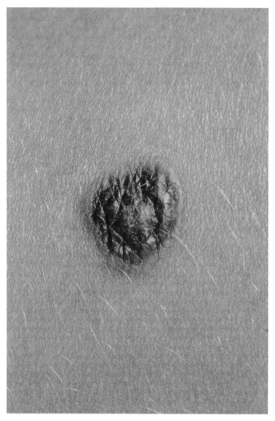

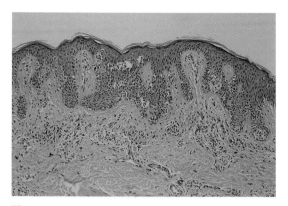

Figure 3.8
Clark's nevus, compound type. This nevus is characterized by nests of melanocytes at the dermoepidermal junction and in a thickened papillary dermis.

Figure 3.7
Clark's nevus. This lesion is benign because it is relatively small, symmetrical and well circumscribed, and its skin markings are preserved. Note a tan rim around a darker centre. These are the clinical features of a very common type of nevus, a 'dysplastic' nevus.

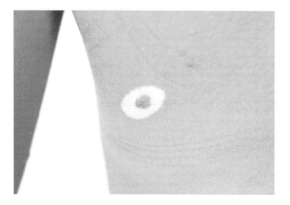

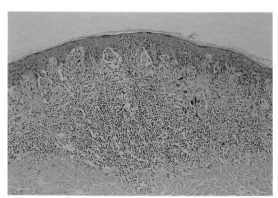

Figure 3.9
Sutton's nevus. In the center, a pigmented Clark's nevus is surrounded by a zone of depigmentation. This constellation of features is that of a 'halo' nevus.

Figure 3.10
Sutton's nevus. This is a Sutton's nevus because of the dense infiltrate of lymphocytes that obscures much of the nevus.

4   ACRODERMATITIS ENTEROPATHICA

Acrodermatitis enteropathica is a rare autosomal-recessive disease caused by a deficiency of zinc. It is characterized by protean signs, including orificial and acral dermatitis, diarrhea and alopecia. These symptoms become evident during infancy by the time the child is weaned.

CLINICAL FINDINGS

The earliest signs of acrodermatitis enteropathica in an infant are lack of interest in feeding, apathy and irritability. Typically, there are crops of vesicles and pustules that often appear around body orifices. In time, these become reddish, psoriasiform plaques covered by scaly crusts (Fig. 4.1). Concurrent with these signs are alopecia of the eyebrows, eyelashes and scalp (Fig. 4.2), severe persistent diarrhea and cachexia. Nail changes include irregular transverse ridges, onychodystrophy, onycholysis and paronychia that becomes chronic. Blepharitis, conjunctivitis and photophobia may also occur.

LABORATORY FINDINGS

Low plasma zinc levels (less than 500 mg/dl) are found in acrodermatitis enteropathica.

HISTOPATHOLOGICAL FINDINGS

Features of well-established lesions are parakeratosis, hypogranulosis, marked ballooning of keratinocytes in the upper part of the epidermis and a sparse, superficial perivascular infiltrate of lymphocytes (Figs 4.3 and 4.4).

ETIOLOGY AND PATHOGENESIS

Acrodermatitis enteropathica results from a poor absorption of zinc from the intestine. The cause of the malabsorption is not yet known. It may be due to an inadequate pancreatic secretion of a ligand that binds to zinc in the intestinal lumen and transports the zinc into the mucosa. The cutaneous and systemic features of the disease are the consequence of the zinc deficiency, since zinc is an indispensable constituent of more than 200 metalloenzymes.

MANAGEMENT

Elemental zinc, 5 mg/kg per day, given as zinc sulfate, zinc gluconate, or zinc dipicolinate, produces a dramatic disappearance of the signs and symptoms of acrodermatitis enteropathica. Diarrhea stops within 1 day. The child's mood improves in 1–2 days. Skin lesions clear in 1–2 weeks. Within 1 month, there is marked improvement in body growth and hair growth.

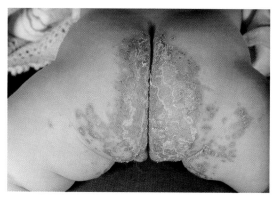

Figure 4.1
Acrodermatitis enteropathica. Discrete violaceous papules and well-circumscribed, brownish plaques are covered by prominent scales and crusts. The lesions are psoriasiform and typically located around body orifices.

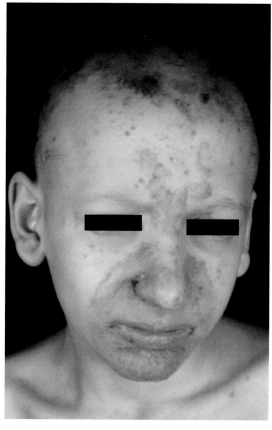

Figure 4.2
Acrodermatitis enteropathica. Pustules, erosions, scales and crusts are present around the nose and the mouth. Note the extensive blepharitis and patchy alopecia.

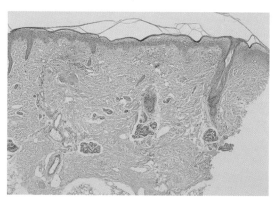

Figure 4.3

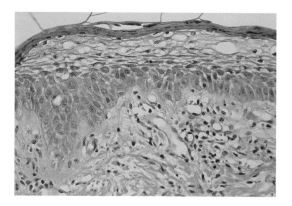

Figure 4.4

Figures 4.3 and 4.4
Acrodermatitis enteropathica. The characteristic features consist of marked ballooning of keratinocytes and slight spongiosis in the upper half of the epidermis, associated with epidermal necrosis. The severe ballooning causes reticular alteration, a net-like appearance of the epidermis formed by membranes of swollen necrotic cells.

ACUTE HEMORRHAGIC EDEMA OF INFANCY

Acute hemorrhagic edema of infancy (AHEI) (Finkelstein's disease) is a distinctive expression of leukocytoclastic vasculitis. It is characterized by tender edema and rosette-shaped purpuric lesions that resolve without treatment.

CLINICAL FINDINGS

The onset of AHEI is acute and marked by fever, exquisitely tender symmetric edematous foci on the face and extremities (Figs 5.1 and 5.2), and, subsequently, the rapid development of a characteristic purpuric eruption within areas of pre-existing edema. Lesions begin as edematous papules with central petechiae that expand centrifugally to form three distinct zones – a central hemorrhagic crust surrounded by a pale palpable annulus which, in turn, is rimmed by redness that blanches on pressure. These rosette-like lesions may become confluent to form purpuric patches and plaques that assume nummular, arciform or polycyclic shapes. Lesions appear in crops and, at any given time, they may be in different stages of development. Sites of predilection are the face, the upper part of the trunk and the arms.

The infant seems to be in great distress and may cry incessantly. Aside from warmth caused by fever and the skin lesions, the physical examination is normal. Despite the impressive lesions, the course is uneventful; and resolution occurs spontaneously in 1–3 weeks, with post-inflammatory pigmentary changes. Recurrences have never been reported.

Age of onset

AHEI is a rare disease of newborns, but children up to 2 years of age may be affected. The disease occurs mostly during winter, after an upper respiratory tract infection.

LABORATORY FINDINGS

Elevated erythrocyte sedimentation rate, leukocytosis (lymphocytic or polymorphonuclear) and elevated alpha-2 globulin may be present. There is no hematuria.

HISTOPATHOLOGICAL FINDINGS

Early in the course of the disease, there is a superficial and deep, perivascular and interstitial infiltrate composed mostly of neutrophils and of abundant nuclear 'dust' (Figs 5.3 and 5.4). Later, the neutrophil infiltrate becomes denser, and deposits of fibrin are present in the walls of some venules. In sum, the histological changes of AHEI are those of leukocytoclastic vasculitis.

ETIOLOGY AND PATHOGENESIS

The cause of AHEI is unknown. The increased frequency of the disease during winter and its association with upper respiratory tract infections (and also vaccinations) suggest that this special expression of leukocytoclastic vasculitis is mediated by immune complexes generated in response to infectious agents.

MANAGEMENT

No treatment is required.

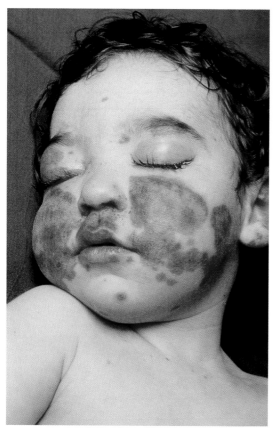

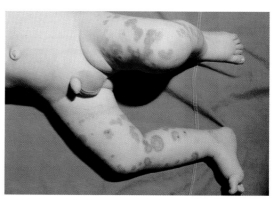

Figure 5.2
Acute hemorrhagic edema of infancy. Rust-colored macules, papules and plaques are present on the legs. Some of the plaques have an arciform configuration, others are arranged in concentric sign and still others have a scalloped appearance. The rust color is a consequence of extravasation of erythrocytes in the upper part of the dermis.

Figure 5.1
Acute hemorrhagic edema of infancy. Papules and plaques with slightly elevated, scalloped borders have a deep red and purple color. The eyelids are edematous.

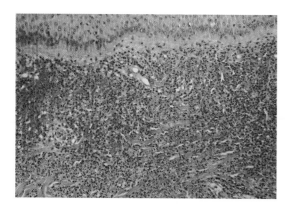

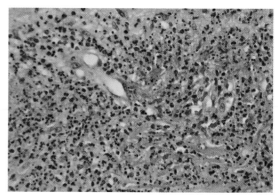

Figure 5.3

Figure 5.4

Figures 5.3 and 5.4
Acute hemorrhagic edema of infancy. Photomicrographs illustrating a fully developed lesion of leukocytoclastic vasculitis.

6 ALOPECIA AREATA

Alopecia areata is a common disorder characterized by well-circumscribed patches of hair loss from any part of the body, but especially from the scalp (Fig. 6.1). If there is loss of hair from the entire scalp, the condition is called alopecia totalis (Fig. 6.2), and is there is loss of hair from the entire body, it is called alopecia universalis. The disease usually begins at about 4–5 years of age. A positive family history is obtained in 10–20% of patients (see Fig. 6.2).

CLINICAL FINDINGS

The onset of alopecia areata is sudden. There are no symptoms other than loss of hair. Lesions consist of well-circumscribed, round or oval patches that are either completely devoid of hair or have little of it. The lesions are usually situated on the scalp, but they may be present on any part of the body that bears hair. The skin in these zones is smooth and, in Caucasians, ivory–white. A feature considered pathognomonic for alopecia areata is 'exclamation point' hairs. These are short stumps of hair that are broad at their distal end and very narrow at their proximal end (hence the analogy to an exclamation point). Exclamation point hairs are found most readily at the margins of lesions.

Alopecia areata may be estimated to be active if, when hairs are pulled at the margin of a lesion, more than five or six hairs come out in one tug. The initial patch of alopecia areata may remain solitary and enlarge centrifugally, or new patches may appear and become confluent.

Ophiasis refers to a clinical form of alopecia areata that occurs mainly in children and consists of a patch of alopecia that begins in the occipital region and extends in a band around the base of the scalp.

When the hair regrows, usually in the center of the patches, new hairs are thin and often white or gray. Recurrences are frequent. Dystrophy of the nail plate is seen in 10–20% of patients.

Associations

Autoimmune diseases such as vitiligo, pernicious anemia, Hashimoto's thyroiditis, diabetes mellitus, and Addison's disease are more common in patients with alopecia areata than in the rest of the population

LABORATORY FINDINGS

There is increased likelihood of detecting thyroid microsomal and thyroglobulin antibodies as well as antibodies against gastric parietal cells and smooth muscle cells in patients with alopecia areata.

HISTOPATHOLOGICAL FINDINGS

Early in the course of alopecia areata there are infiltrates of lymphocytes around hair follicle bulbs in the anagenic phase. Later, whorls of collagen bundles that contain degenerated glassy membranes appear at sites where follicular papillae have been bared during catagen or at its onset (Figs 6.3 and 6.4).

ETIOLOGY AND PATHOGENESIS

The cause of alopecia areata is not known. The increased incidence of autoimmune disorders in association with alopecia areata suggests that it is an autoimmune disease sustained by antibodies against the hair bulbs.

MANAGEMENT

No curative treatments are currently available. The most popular agents for management of alopecia areata are corticosteroids. Children with very localized alopecia can be treated with topical corticosteroids applied twice a day. Intralesional injections must be avoided. If there is no response to this therapy or the disease is widespread, an induction of allergic contact dermatitis with diphencyprone or squaric acid dibutylester may be attempted. Psychotherapy may be a very important support.

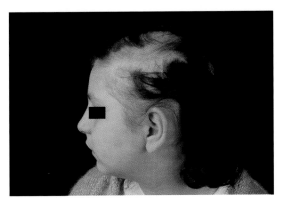

Figure 6.1
Alopecia areata. Patches have become confluent as a consequence of extreme involvement of the scalp. The circular patch of the occiput helps to differentiate this condition from trichotillomania. Note that the eyelashes and eyebrows are present.

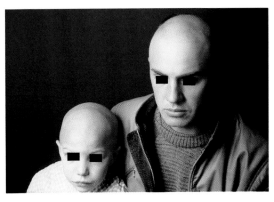

Figure 6.2
Familial alopecia totalis. All the hairs are missing from the scalp of this father and son. The eyebrows are present in both, but the eyelashes are missing in the son.

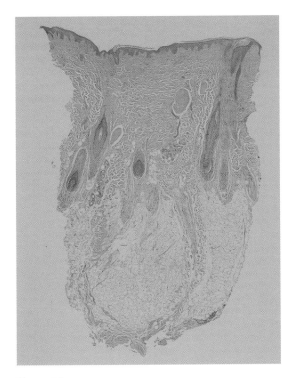

Figure 6.3

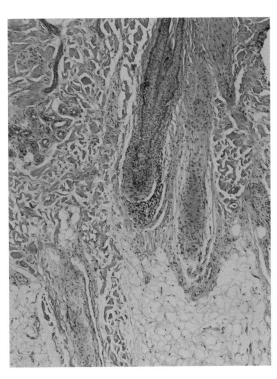

Figure 6.4

Figures 6.3 and 6.4
Alopecia areata. There are hair follicles in both anagen and catagen. The follicles are thinned and situated wholly in the dermis rather than rooted in the normal position for follicles on the scalp, namely in the subcutaneous fat. Fibrous tracts are present beneath the follicles in catagen, and a moderately dense lymphohistiocytic infiltrate is present around the bulbs. The latter is a *sine qua non* for diagnosis of active lesions of alopecia areata.

7 ANETODERMA

Anetoderma is a specific type of cutaneous atrophy that develops secondary to inflammatory processes. It is marked by circumscribed areas of thin, soft, wrinkled skin that usually bulge above the regular surface of the skin, although they may be slightly depressed (Fig. 7.1).

EPIDEMIOLOGY

Anetoderma is rare and may be familial. The onset is usually in the first or second decade of life.

CLINICAL FINDINGS

The typical lesions vary in size from less than 1 mm to a few centimeters (see Figs 7.1, 7.2). The number, site and distribution of the lesions depend on the nature of the primary process. The sites most commonly involved are the arms, the neck, the chest and the upper part of the back. The atrophic skin does not ulcerate. Anetoderma persists once it has developed.

HISTOPATHOLOGICAL FINDINGS

The dominant pathological findings are a focal alteration and loss of collagen (Fig. 7.3) and the absence of elastic fibers (Fig. 7.4) in the middle and upper parts of the reticular dermis.

ETIOLOGY AND PATHOGENESIS

Anetoderma is an end-stage of a variety of disorders that cause loss of collagen and elastic tissue. Release of enzymes from inflammatory cells seems to be the common denominator for development of this distinct form of atrophy. Acne vulgaris and varicella are the most frequent causes of anetoderma in children.

MANAGEMENT

No treatment has been successful.

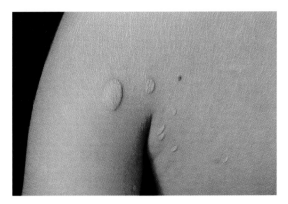

Figure 7.1
Anetoderma. These skin-colored papules and plaques are herniated easily into the subcutaneous fat by slight pressure. This process doubtlessly began as an inflammation, but its precise nature cannot be defined.

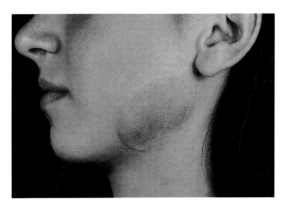

Figure 7.2
Anetoderma. This sagging plaque fulfils the criteria for cutaneous atrophy because the skin wrinkles easily in both the hypopigmented and the hyperpigmented areas, and it is covered by numerous telangiectases. An atrophic lesion such as this was once a long-standing inflammatory plaque.

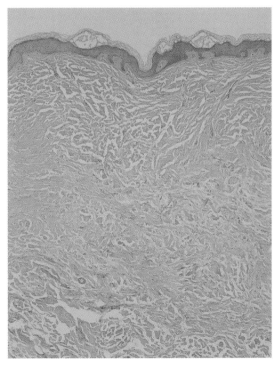

Figure 7.3
Anetoderma. The collagen in the middle part of the reticular dermis is different from the normal skin in terms of thickness and orientation. The collagen bundles are thinner and less parallel to the skin surface. (Hematoxylin and eosin stain.)

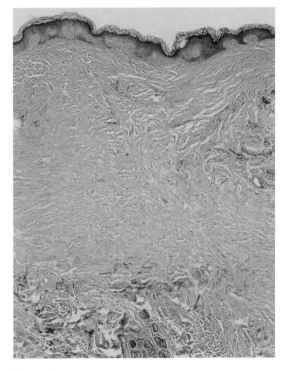

Figure 7.3
Anetoderma. This section stained with elastic tissue stain confirms that the abnormal zone is in the middle part of the reticular dermis, where the elastic fibers are markedly decreased in number.

ANGIOBLASTOMA

Cutaneous angioblastoma of Nakagawa is a rare, benign, vascular neoplasm composed mostly of immature endothelial cells.

EPIDEMIOLOGY

Angioblastoma is an uncommon tumor that chiefly affects prepubertal children.

CLINICAL FINDINGS

The earliest sign of angioblastoma is a poorly demarcated pink or red macule or patch. This soon evolves into a deep red, blue or purple indurated plaque (Fig. 8.1) or a cluster of nodules and tumors of similar color. Lesions are often painful. Tenderness is acknowledged by about 90% of patients. The neoplasm is almost always solitary, and the sites of predilection, in descending order of frequency, are the neck, trunk, extremities and head. The neoplasm neither metastasizes nor regresses without treatment, but it usually persists. The well-being of the patient is unaffected.

HISTOPATHOLOGICAL FINDINGS

Lobules of plump oval cells are aligned along pre-existing vascular plexuses in the dermis and sometimes in the subcutaneous fat. Many of these cells surround tiny lumina of vessels that resemble capillaries (Figs. 8.2 and 8.3).

MANAGEMENT

Complete surgical excision is the best treatment. Therapy with soft X-rays has also been reported to be effective.

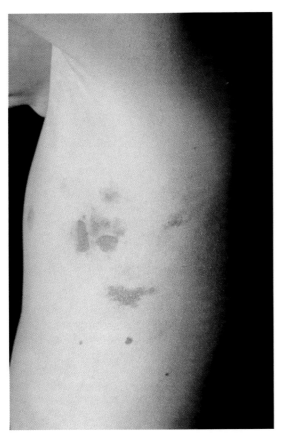

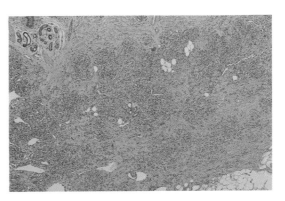

Figure 8.2

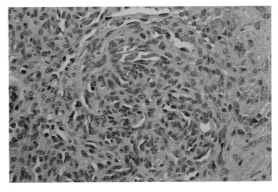

Figure 8.3

Figure 8.1
Angioblastoma. Numerous red plaques of various sizes with shapes and scalloped borders can be seen.

Figures 8.2 and 8.3
Angioblastoma. In the lower half of the dermis and in the upper part of subcutaneous fat there are clusters of numerous, closely crowded, small blood vessels lined by plump oval endothelial cells.

9   ANGIOKERATOMA

Angiokeratomas are vascular lesions with keratotic elements. They appear clinically as dark red to black papules covered by scales. Angiokeratomas may be subdivided into localized types (angiokeratoma of Mibelli, angiokeratoma of Fordyce, angiokeratoma circumscriptum) and widespread types (Fabry's disease).

CLINICAL FINDINGS

Angiokeratoma of Mibelli consists of typical red to purple, keratotic, asymptomatic papules of 2–5 mm diameter, situated over bony prominences such as the dorsa of fingers and toes (Fig. 9.l), elbows and knees. This rare type of angiokeratoma begins in childhood or early adolescence and persists for life. It occurs mostly in females.

Angiokeratoma of Fordyce is the commonest of all the angiokeratomas. It is characterized by dome-shaped reddish–purple papules of 2–4 mm in diameter, situated on the scrotum (Fig. 9.2) or vulva. If traumatized, angiokeratomas of Fordyce may bleed profusely because the venules that they comprise are superficial.

Angiokeratoma circumscriptum is the least common type of all the angiokeratomas. It presents as a large, solitary, linear, unilateral plaque composed of verrucous dark red to black papules that have become confluent (Fig. 9.3). Half of the lesions reported on have had their onset in infancy, and some were present at birth. With age, angiokeratoma circumscriptum tends to increase in size and become increasingly keratotic. There is no tendency to involution.

Angiokeratoma corporis diffusum (Fabry's disease) is a rare genetic disorder transmitted in an X-linked fashion. It results from an inborn error of glycophingolipid metabolism caused by a deficiency of alphagalactosidase A, which leads to an accumulation of uncatabolized ceramide in all tissues and cells of the body. Skin lesions begin to erupt before puberty and consist of numerous, tiny, dark red, punctuate papules (Fig. 9.4) that occur in clusters distributed symmetrically on the buttock and thighs. In males, important symptoms related to involvement of other organs are excruciating episodic crises of acral pain (Fabry's crises), acral paresthesias, transient ischemic attacks, systemic thrombosis, destructive corneal dystrophy and progressive renal failure that ultimately causes death. The diagnosis is confirmed from decreased plasma levels of alphagalactosidase A.

HISTOPATHOLOGICAL FINDINGS

The common denominators of the angiokeratomas (Fig. 9.5) are:

- focal compact orthokeratosis of variable degree;
- widely dilated, thin-walled, endothelium-lined blood vessels in the upper part of the dermis;
- a thin zone of collagen that separates the dilated blood vessels from the epidermis.

MANAGEMENT

Angiokeratomas may be treated by laser, cryosurgery, electrodesiccation with curettage, or surgical excision.

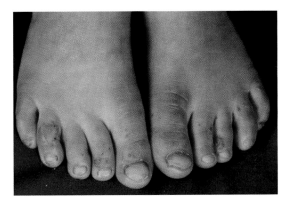

Figure 9.1
Angiokeratoma of Mibelli. Discrete reddish papules are situated on the toes. Some of the papules have become confluent and formed plaques.

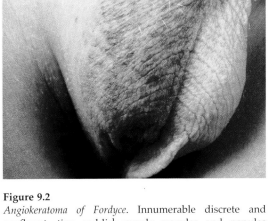

Figure 9.2
Angiokeratoma of Fordyce. Innumerable discrete and confluent, tiny reddish–purple macules and papules cover half of the scrotum.

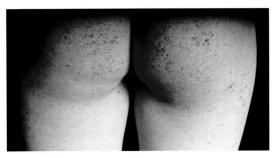

Figure 9.4
Angiokeratoma corporis diffusum (Fabry's disease). The buttocks are covered with rust colored and red–black macules and papules, each of which is an individual angiokeratoma. The distribution of lesions is typical.

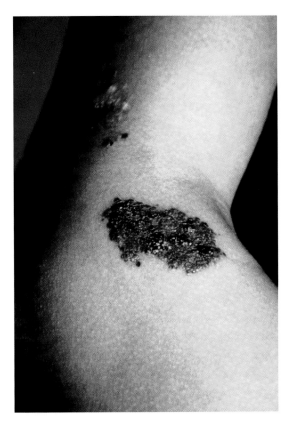

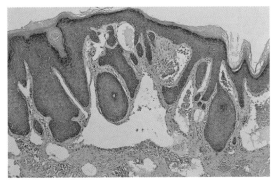

Figure 9.3
Angiokeratoma circumscriptum. This multicolored plaque has scalloped borders and is studded with pink, purple and black papules covered by scales. The combination of vascular proliferation and scales makes this an angiokeratoma.

Figure 9.5
Angiokeratoma. The neoplasm is well circumscribed and is composed of widely dilated, blood-filled vessels. The epidermis is focally hyperplastic, hypergranulotic and hyperkeratotic.

10 ANGIOLYMPHOID HYPERPLASIA

Angiolymphoid hyperplasia is a distinctive vascular disorder that results from an arteriovenous shunt. It is often accompanied by infiltrates of lymphocytes and eosinophils.

EPIDEMIOLOGY

The condition may occur in young children and adolescents. Three-quarters of the patients are female.

CLINICAL FINDINGS

Angiolymphoid hyperplasia may consist of a single lesion (as it does in 80% of patients) or of many lesions. The lesions are dome-shaped, shiny, pink, purple or reddish–brown papules and nodules (Fig. 10.1), that are most commonly situated on the face, especially around the ears, and on the scalp. The lesions tend to persist. The general health of the patient is unaffected.

LABORATORY FINDINGS

Peripheral eosinophilia is present in less than 20% of patients.

HISTOPATHOLOGICAL FINDINGS

The lesion is well circumscribed and consists of widely dilated, thick-walled blood vessels lined by plump endothelial cells that protrude prominently into the lumens (Figs 10.2 and 10.3). Inflammatory cells (mostly lymphocytes) are nearly always present in the dermis.

ETIOLOGY AND PATHOGENESIS

The cause is not known.

MANAGEMENT

Injection of corticosteroids directly into lesions may be beneficial by causing them to resolve at least partially. If that fails, surgical excision is the treatment of choice. Other modalities, including cryotherapy, radiation therapy and laser therapy, have not been successful.

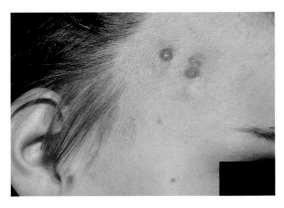

Figure 10.1
Angiolymphoid hyperplasia. Well-circumscribed, smooth-surfaced, pink–orange papules situated on the face.

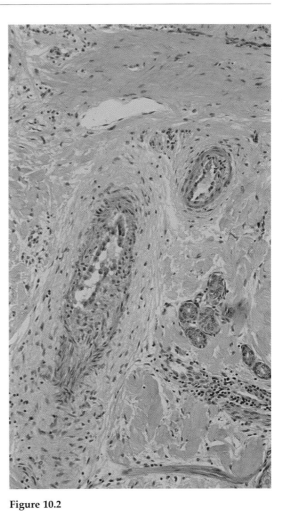

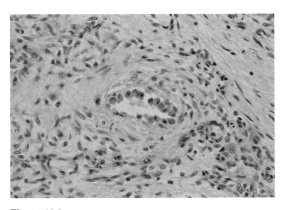

Figure 10.3

Figure 10.2

Figures 10.2 and 10.3
Angiolymphoid hyperplasia. Throughout the dermis there is an increased number of widely dilated, thick-walled blood vessels. Endothelial cells protrude far into the lumens.

APLASIA CUTIS CONGENITA

Aplasia cutis congenita is a localized absence of skin. It is present at birth and occurs in about 1 in 10,000 newborns.

CLINICAL FINDINGS

Aplasia cutis congenita consists at first of one or more well-circumscribed ulcers with granulation tissue at the base (Fig. 11.1). The individual lesions may be round, oval or triangular. The commonest site is the midline of the scalp, usually near the vertex. The second commonest site is a lower limb. Any site, however, may be involved. Upon healing, defects are replaced by smooth white, gray or yellowish scars (Fig. 11.2).

Associations

Aplasia cutis congenita may be found in association with other developmental defects.

HISTOPATHOLOGICAL FINDINGS

Aplasia cutis congenita consists of ulcers that involve the dermis and sometimes the subcutaneous fat. The ulcers heal with scarring.

ETIOLOGY AND PATHOGENESIS

The cause of this disorder has yet to be established. Various factors, such as intrauterine injury, effects of a drug and viral diseases in the mother, have been implicated, but none has been proven to be a cause.

MANAGEMENT

Every attempt should be made to avoid trauma to the involved site. Local cleanliness can prevent secondary infection. If there is neither trauma nor secondary infection, the defects of the skin and of the underlying skull should heal in a few months.

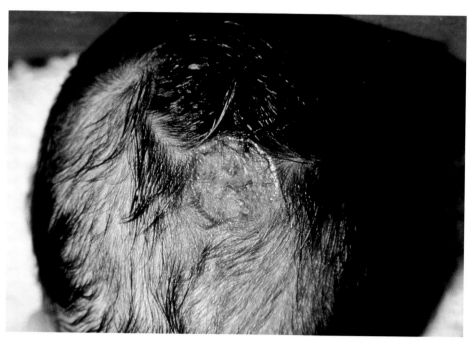

Figure 11.1
Aplasia cutis congenita. In a newborn, there is a round, sharply marginated ulcer surrounded by an elevated border.

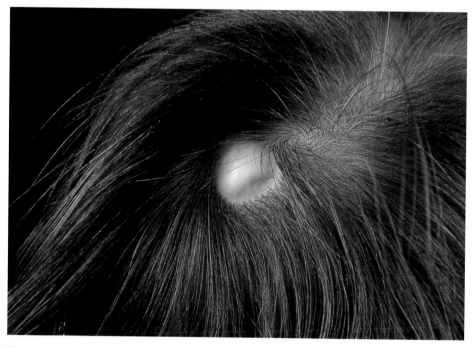

Figure 11.2
Aplasia cutis congenita. This smooth alopecic yellow–white scar can be determined to be long-standing because of these features and also because of the absence of pinkness.

12   ASYMMETRICAL PERIFLEXURAL EXANTHEM OF CHILDHOOD

Asymmetrical periflexural exanthem of childhood is an exanthem of unknown etiology that typically involves one axillary fold with central spread – this explains the term 'unilateral laterothoracic exanthem of childhood', which is used by some authors.

CLINICAL FINDINGS

Asymmetrical periflexural exanthem of childhood appears as either a maculopapular scarlatiniform eruption or an eczematiform dermatitis that involves one axillary fold and spreads centrally on to the thorax and proximal part of the corresponding arm (Figs 12.1 and 12.2). In a minority of patients, initial lesions develop around the antecubital or popliteal flexures; onset around distal flexures or on the face is rare.

The lesions tend to be confluent around the fold and become more sparse distally. Individual lesions can be purpuric. After 5–10 days, similar but smaller lesions appear on the contralateral side, and rarely the exanthem becomes more diffuse, with minor lesions elsewhere. The disease does not affect the general health but can be moderately pruriginous. Mild ipsilateral lymphadenopathy can be found in about 50% of cases.

Resolution with mild hyperpigmentation or pityriasis desquamation is noted in about 1 month.

The age of the patients is typically between the ages of 1 and 4 years, although adults can also be affected. The presence of small epidemics has been noted, and the condition is often associated with prodromal symptoms of an upper respiratory tract or digestive tract infection.

HISTOPATHOLOGICAL FINDINGS

Skin biopsy usually is non-contributory. Histology is non-specific, showing areas of epidermal spongiosis accompanied by exocytosis of mononuclear cells, while a moderate perivascular and periappendageal lymphohistiocytic infiltrate is present in the dermis.

ETIOLOGY AND PATHOGENESIS

The cause of asymmetrical periflexural exanthem of childhood is presently unknown. However, the features in favor of a viral origin for the condition are numerous – the age of the patients, the presence of small epidemics, the frequency of associated prodromes, the spontaneous resolution in a few weeks, the regional lymphadenopathy, the lack of response to antibiotics and topical corticosteroids. The possible causative role of parvovirus B19 is anecdotal.

MANAGEMENT

Treatment is not necessary is most instances. Symptomatic oral antihistamines and non-steroidal lenitive creams can be prescribed when necessary. Topical corticosteroids are not effective.

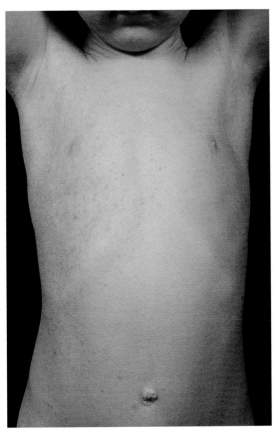

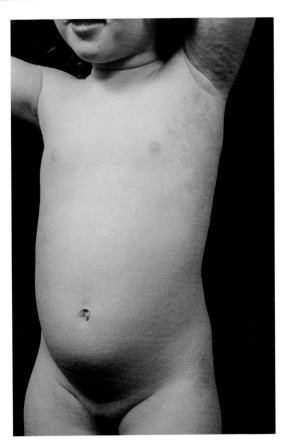

Figure 12.1

Asymmetrical periflexural exanthem of childhood. A maculopapular scarlatiniform eruption involves the right axillary fold of this child, with spread on to the thorax and proximal inner part of the correspinding arm. A cluster of lesions is also present on the hip.

Figure 12.2

Asymmetrical periflexural exanthem of childhood. In this infant the rash is more eczematiform and involves the left side of the body. It affects the same sites as the patient shown in Fig. 12.1.

ATOPIC DERMATITIS

Atopic dermatitis is a disease of children with personal or family histories of allergic urticaria, allergic rhinitis or allergic asthma. It results from severely pruritic skin.

EPIDEMIOLOGY

Atopic dermatitis is a common disorder that affects about 3% of all infants. Symptoms of the disease may be noted shortly after birth and they appear by the first year in 60% of patients.

CLINICAL FINDINGS

Findings in atopic dermatitis vary with age. Acute skin lesions consist of erythematous patches of intensely pruritic papules and hints of vesicles that ooze and become crusted (Figs 13.1, 13.2 and 13.3). These lesions may appear first on the face, with sparing of the perioral and perinasal skin (see Fig. 13.1); later the extremities, dorsa of the hands (see Fig. 13.2) and flexures (see Fig. 13.3) are involved.

Chronic skin lesions consist of thickening of the skin with accentuation of skin markings (lichenification) as a consequence of persistent rubbing (Figs 13.4, 13.5 and 13.6). These lesions usually affect children over the age of 3 years. They often involve the popliteal and antecubital fossae, the ankles, the wrists and the sides of the neck.

Stigmata of atopic dermatitis include dry skin and characteristic creases on the lower eyelids (Dennie–Morgan sign). Special features are represented by pityriasis alba and juvenile plantar dermatosis. Pityriasis alba is characterized by several round, asymptomatic, hypopigmented patches covered by subtle scales. These patches are mainly confined to the face and limbs (Fig. 13.7). Juvenile plantar dermatosis is characterized by redness, scaling and painful fissures on weight-bearing parts of the feet (Fig 13.8).

Atopic dermatitis is long-lasting with exacerbations and remissions. A spontaneous, more or less complete remission during childhood is the rule.

Associations

Asthma and allergic rhinitis occur in about 30% of patients, cataract in 10%, ichthyosis vulgaris and keratosis pilaris in 5%. Alopecia areata and defective polymorphonuclear chemotactic activity each occur in less than 1% of patients.

COMPLICATIONS

The most common complication is secondary infection by *Staphylococcus aureus* and herpes simplex virus (eczema herpeticum).

LABORATORY FINDINGS

Between 60 and 70% of patients with atopic dermatitis have elevated serum levels of immunoglobulin E. About 40% have hypereosinophilia. A few have a deficiency of T lymphocytes.

HISTOPATHOLOGICAL FINDINGS

In very early lesions, intraepidermal intercellular edema, spongiosis are seen (Fig. 13.9). Later, characteristic features of lichen simplex chronicus (hyperkeratosis, hypergranulosis, irregular acanthosis and dermal lymphohistiocytic infiltrate) appear (Fig. 13.10).

ETIOLOGY AND PATHOGENESIS

The cause of atopic dermatitis is unknown. Elevated levels of serum immunoglobulin E and the fact that these tend to correlate with the severity of atopic dermatitis have been interpreted to suggest that hypersensitivity reactions may be responsible for most of the manifestations of the disease. It has been demonstrated that epidermal Langerhans cells possess high-affinity immunoglobulin E receptors, through which eczema-like reaction could be triggered.

MANAGEMENT

The single most important step in management of atopic dermatitis is prevention of pruritus. Educating the patient to avoid rubbing and scratching, to prevent dry skin and to wear cotton clothes is very important. Treatments that are helpful in managing pruritus and inflammatory lesions of atopic dermatitis include:

- oral antihistamines for pruritus;
- oral antibiotics to cure staphylococcal infections;
- topical emollients to prevent xerosis;
- topical non-steroidal anti-inflammatory agents, which may be the treatment of choice;
- topical corticosteroids when necessary (long-term use must be avoided);
- ultraviolet B and ultraviolet A phototherapy, which may be effective;
- systemic corticosteroids, or cyclosporin, which should be reserved for patients with important life-threatening problems and used only for short courses.

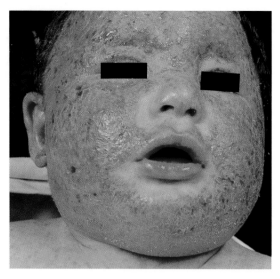

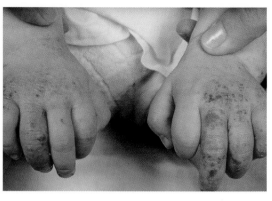

Figure 13.1
Atopic dermatitis. Weeping lesions are eroded and crusted. The crusts are both serous and hemorrhagic. Observe the sparing of the skin around the nose and the lower lip.

Figure 13.2
Atopic dermatitis. There are many erosions, hemorrhagic crusts and lichenified papules. Hemorrhagic crusts are the consequence of vigorous scratching, and lichenified papules are the result of persistent rubbing.

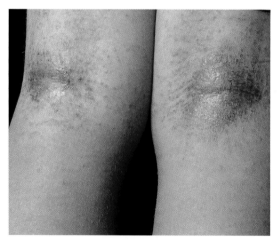

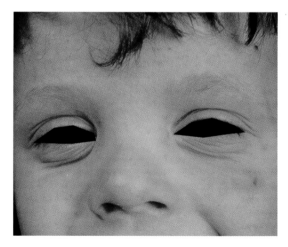

Figure 13.3
Atopic dermatitis. Numerous eroded papules in the popliteal fossa have become confluent. These lesions have been secondarily denuded by vigorous scratching.

Figure 13.4
Atopic dermatitis. The periorbital skin of both eyelids is markedly thickened, reddish and scaly. The skin markings of the lower eyelids are accentuated and the eyebrows are partially alopecic. These changes do not develop spontaneously but are the consequence of prolonged external trauma.

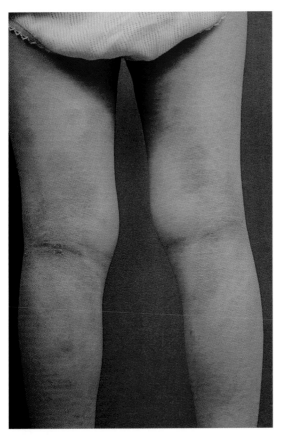

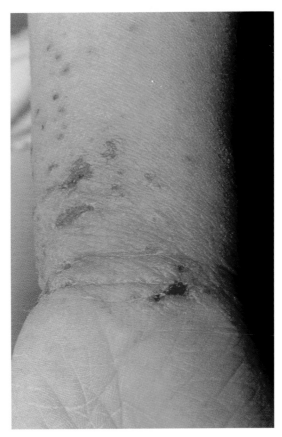

Figure 13.5
Atopic dermatitis. Popliteal fossae are a site of predilection in children over 3 years of age.

Figure 13.6
Atopic dermatitis. Hemorrhagic crusts, ulcerations and erosions are the consequence of vigorous scratching, and lichenification is the result of persistent rubbing.

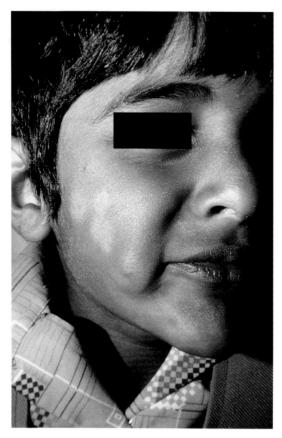

Figure 13.7
Pityriasis alba. The hypopigmented nummular lesions in this Indian boy represent post-inflammatory hypopigmentation.

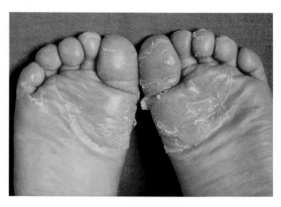

Figure 13.8
Juvenile plantar dermatosis. This term is given to scales on top of shiny skin in the area affected by atopic dermatitis. Symmetrical lesions such as these could conceivably be a manifestation of atopic dermatitis, but this a mere supposition.

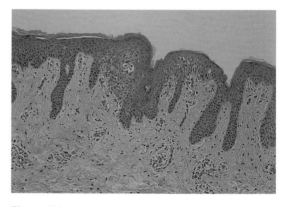

Figure 13.9
Atopic dermatitis. Foci of spongiosis are evident within the epidermis.

Figure 13.10
Atopic dermatitis. Lichen simplex chronicus. The indubitable signs of chronic persistent rubbing are seen here. These signs are orthokeratosis, hypergranulosis, irregular acanthosis and dermal lymphohistiocytic infiltration.

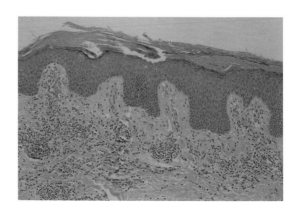

Basal cell carcinoma is a poorly differentiated malignant neoplasm composed of basaloid cells that arise from basal cells of the epidermis or epithelial structures of adnexa. Basal cell carcinoma is extremely rare in children and may be either a solitary neoplasm or one of numerous neoplasms in the nevoid–basal cell carcinoma syndrome.

SOLITARY BASAL CELL CARCINOMA

CLINICAL FINDINGS

Basal cell carcinomas in children have the same clinical features as in adults. They evolve as smooth, skin-colored or opalescent, shiny, roundish, asymptomatic papules that in time may develop rolled margins covered by telangiectases and central ulcers (Fig. 14.1). The neoplasms vary in size from millimeters to many centimeters in greatest diameter. Sites of predilection are the face, particularly the nose, cheeks and eyelids, the neck and the shoulders. The trunk and extremities may also be involved.

Various morphological expressions of basal cell carcinomas seen in adults are also noted in children (i.e. superficial, nodular, ulceronodular, pigmented, fibroepithelial, adenoid, adenoid cystic, and sclerodermoid or morpheiform) (Fig. 14.2). These tumors are mostly seen in the second decade of life.

HISTOPATHOLOGICAL FINDINGS

Basal cell carcinomas are characterized by asymmetrical aggregations of basaloid cells.

The peripheral cells of these aggregations are arranged in palisades and are separated from the surrounding altered stroma by clefts (Figs 14.5 and 14.6).

ETIOLOGY AND PATHOGENESIS

No cause is known for basal cell carcinomas in children who have received little exposure to sunlight.

MANAGEMENT

Surgical excision is the treatment of choice. Mohs surgery is indicated in certain locations, such as the central area of the face and around the ears. Small lesions can be treated with laser therapy or electrosurgery.

NEVOID–BASAL CELL CARCINOMA SYNDROME

Nevoid–basal cell carcinoma syndrome (NBCS) is a genetic disorder characterized by numerous basal cell carcinomas, pits in the palms of the hand and soles of the feet, cysts in the jaw, skeletal anomalies and ectopic calcifications.

EPIDEMIOLOGY

NBCS has an autosomal-dominant inheritance. It usually begins during childhood.

CLINICAL FINDINGS

Children afflicted with NBCS develop numerous basal cell carcinomas, which appear as translucent skin-colored or pigmented papules and nodules with or without ulcers (Figs 14.3 and 14.4). The lesions are located on the face, neck and upper trunk. In addition, 60% of patients have numerous irregularly shaped pits, 1–3 mm in diameter, on the palms and of the hands and the soles of the feet. Patients continue to develop basal cell carcinomas with increasing frequency throughout life.

Associations

Among the more common anomalies associated with the NBCS are skeletal defects such as cysts of the jaws (in 80% of patients), neural defects such as calcification of the falx cerebri (in 80%), anomalies of the vertebrae (in 65%), abnormalities of the ribs (in 60%) and cysts of the long bones and phalanges (in 45%). Ophthalmological defects include hypertelorism (in 30% of patients), strabis-mus (in 25%), and congenital blindness (in 5%).

HISTOPATHOLOGICAL FINDINGS

The basal cell carcinomas seen in the NBCS seem to be virtually identical histopathologically to nearly all varieties of solitary basal cell carcinomas described above (Figs 14.5 and 14.6).

ETIOLOGY AND PATHOGENESIS

The cause of NBCS is not known.

MANAGEMENT

Because basal cell carcinomas in NBCS are usually so numerous and tend to behave in a benign manner, not every basal cell carcinoma must be removed. Palmar and plantar pits do not require treatment as long as there is no clinical evidence of carcinoma at those sites.

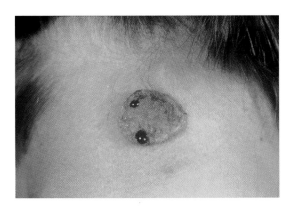

Figure 14.1
Basal cell carcinoma. Sharply circumscribed elevated borders characterize this lesion in a 14-year-old girl. Note the central ulcer covered by blood and crusts.

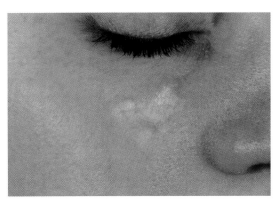

Figure 14.2
Morpheiform basal cell carcinoma. White zones surrounded by pink rims characterize this irregularly shaped plaque. A lesion such as this is exceptional in an adolescent.

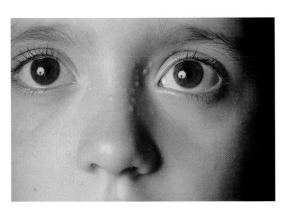

Figure 14.3
Nevoid–basal cell carcinoma syndrome. Each skin-colored papule shown here is a basal cell carcinoma. The face is a site of predilection.

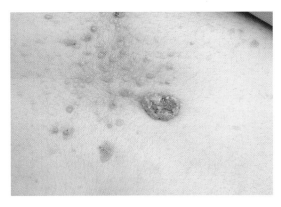

Figure 14.4
Nevoid–basal cell carcinoma syndrome. Basal cell carcinoma in a patient with NBCS. The lesions consist of sharply elevated borders and an ulcer covered by a hemorrhagic crust in the center. Around this lesion there are numerous skin-colored smaller lesions evolving into basal cell carcinomas.

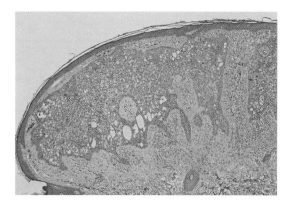

Figure 14.5

Figures 14.5 and 14.6
Nevoid–basal cell carcinoma syndrome. The neoplasm consists of basaloid cells with cribriform and cystic arrangements separated by clefts from the surrounding dermis.

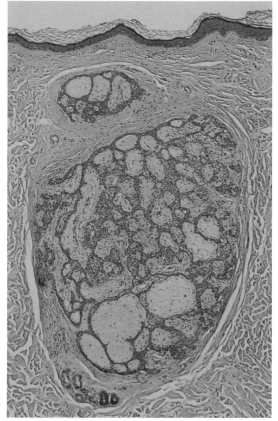

Figure 14.6

15 BECKER'S NEVUS

Becker's nevus is a cutaneous hamartoma that manifests itself clinically as a unilateral hyper-pigmented patch covered more or less by coarse dark hairs.

EPIDEMIOLOGY

Becker's nevus is a common condition. It is more common in boys than girls. It usually appears in the first decade of life.

CLINICAL FINDINGS

Becker's nevus usually consists of a unilateral, localized, brownish patch or a plaque that is so slightly elevated that it is barely discernible. The color ranges from tan to dark brown and is usually uniform except at the periphery, where it may be uneven. The outline is irregular, but the margins are sharply circumscribed. The sites of predilection are the shoulders (Fig. 15.1), the anterior chest and the scapular region. A patch may be as large as 200 mm or more in greatest diameter. In time, sometimes as long as 2 years after onset, hypertrichosis develops in over half of cases. The hairs in the patch are coarser and darker than those on other parts of the body. Few other changes occur to the lesion during the patient's life. The lesion is totally benign.

HISTOPATHOLOGICAL FINDINGS

The epidermis is hyperpigmented with oblong rete ridges that have a flat base. There is an increase number of terminal hair follicles and an increased number of muscles of hair erection (Fig 15.2)

MANAGEMENT

Excision is usually not possible because the lesion is too large. Some patients elect to have the hairs within the lesion removed by laser therapy or electroepilation.

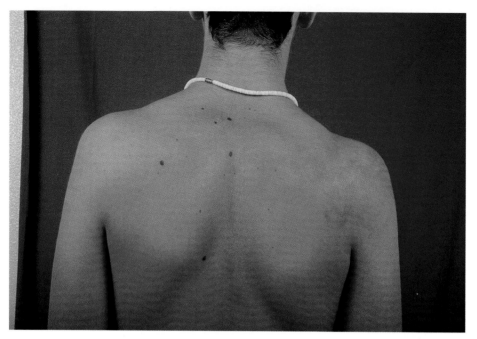

Figure 15.1
Becker's nevus. This browinsh patch covered by hairs is typical. Note the ill-defined borders of the lesion. The shoulder is a site of predilection.

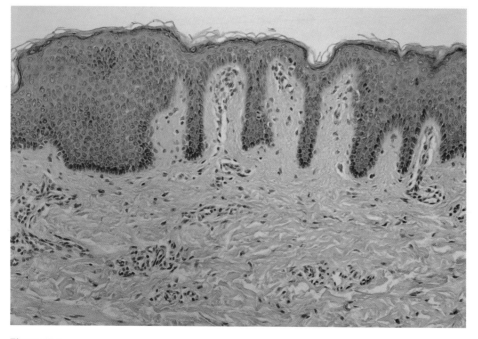

Figure 15.2
Becker's nevus. The lesion can be seen to be a Becker's nevus because the hyperpigmented rete ridges are elongated and some of them have a flattish bottom. Moreover, two terminal hair follicles are in close proximity.

16 BENIGN CEPHALIC HISTIOCYTOSIS

Benign cephalic histiocytosis (BCH) is a self-healing, non-Langerhans cell, non-lipid, cutaneous histiocytosis of children. It usually involves the head.

CLINICAL FINDINGS

BCH begins during the first 3 years of life as an eruption of asymptomatic, yellow to red–brown macules or papules, 2–5 mm in diameter (Figs 16.1 and 16.2). The initial number of lesions varies considerably from a few to more than 100. The individual lesions are slightly raised or flat-topped. The lesions are situated first on the upper part of the face. In time, papules come to cover the entire head and the neck. A few papules may appear on the arms and shoulders and, uncommonly, on the buttocks and thighs. The mucous membranes, palms and soles, and viscera are spared. Spontaneous regression occurs on average 2 years after the onset.

HISTOPATHOLOGICAL FINDINGS

Papules consist of well-circumscribed lymphohistiocytic infiltrates situated immediately beneath the epidermis (Fig. 16.3). Most of the histiocytes have pleomorphic nuclei and abundant, pale, eosinophilic cytoplasm (Fig. 16.4). The histiocytes are S100- and CD1a- and do not contain Langerhans granules

MANAGEMENT

No treatment is necessary because the disease is benign and self-limiting.

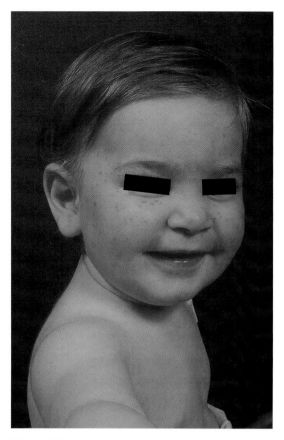

Figure 16.1
Benign cephalic histiocytosis. The papular eruption involves the face exclusively.

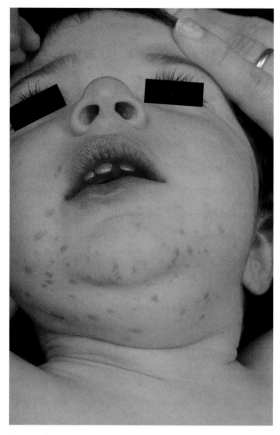

Figure 16.2
Benign cephalic histiocytosis. Many brownish papules are scattered beneath the chin and the cheeks, and most of them are discrete.

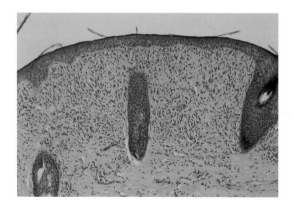

Figure 16.3

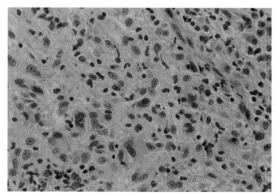

Figure 16.4

Figures 16.3 and 16.4
Benign cephalic histiocytosis. This domed lesion is characterized by a dense diffuse infiltrate of histiocytes, many of them with abundant, pale, eosinophilic cytoplasm.

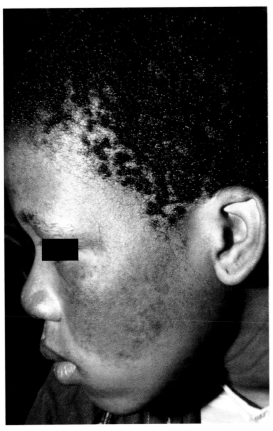

Figure 18.1
Nevus of Ota with scleral involvement. The broad blue–gray patch pictured here is mottled and extends into the sclera.

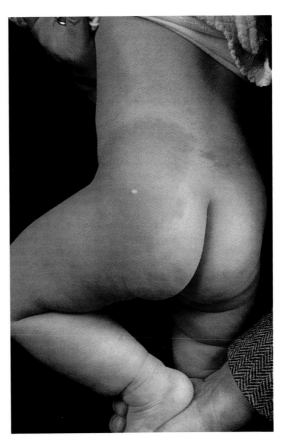

Figure 18.3
Mongolian spot. This lesion on the thigh, buttock and waist is analogous to a nevus of Ota. A Mongolian spot such as the one shown here tends to lighten with time.

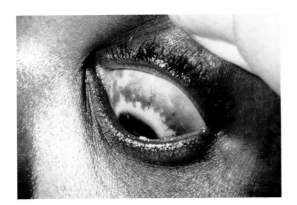

Figure 18.2
Nevus of Ota with scleral involvement. The sceral changes of nevus of Ota are analogous to those in the skin, namely, those of a patch of blue nevus.

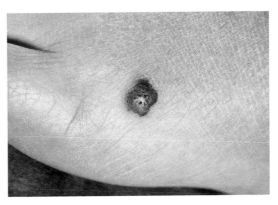

Figure 18.4
Blue nevus. This lesion is benign because is small and well circumscribed; it is a blue nevus because of its bluish hue.

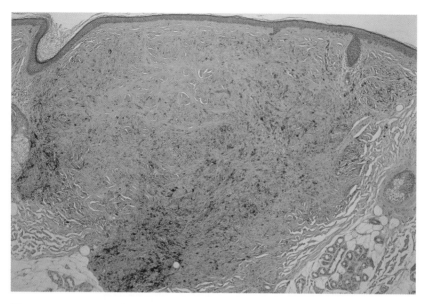

Figure 18.5

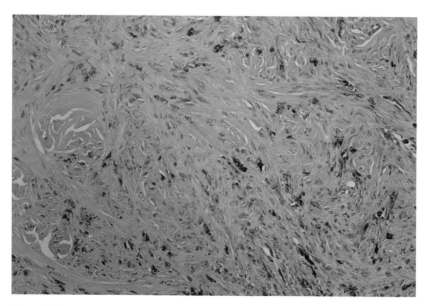

Figure 18.6

Figures 18.5 and 18.6

Blue nevus with collagenization. This relatively small, well-circumscribed lesion fills the dermis and extends into the subcutaneous fat. It is characterized by a proliferation of dendritic and oval-shaped melanocytes. There are also numerous melanophages in addition to melanocytes. The lesions look blue clinically because melanin is present in melanocytes, and collagen bundles are markedly thickened. The latter phenomenon, collagenization, occurs in blue nevi when dendritic melanocytes are scattered among bundles of collagens, and never when they are arranged cohesively in parallel. In papular nevi, dendritic melanocytes are scattered among bundles of collagen and never arranged cohesively in parallel.

19 BLUE RUBBER-BLEB NEVUS SYNDROME

The blue rubber-bleb nevus syndrome (Bean syndrome) is a peculiar angiomatosis characterized by numerous cavern-like hemangiomas that involve the skin, mucous membranes and other parts of the body.

EPIDEMIOLOGY

The syndrome is rare and not usually familial. There is also no predilection for any race or either sex.

CLINICAL FINDINGS

Typical skin lesions of blue rubber-bleb nevus syndrome consist of soft, blue papules that resemble rubber nipples (Fig. 19.1). The lesions are often detected at birth or in early infancy. They are easily compressible and refill promptly when the pressure is released. The lesions often are multiple, sometimes numbering hundreds, and are scattered randomly on the trunk and limbs. The blebs can be painful, both when pressed and without pressure. The pain in these hemangiomas becomes manifest at puberty and is said by patients to be most troublesome at night. In about 90% of patients, numerous hemangiomas are also found in the gastrointestinal tract, most commonly in the small bowel. Lesions may be situated on mucous membranes of the lips, oral cavity (Fig. 19.2), glans penis and nasopharynx. The lungs, urinary tract, liver, spleen, brain, meninges, and heart may be involved by the angiomatosis, although this is rare. New lesions may appear and old ones may continue to grow well into adulthood. The lesions are persistent and prognosis depends on severity of complications.

Complications

Angiomas in the gastrointestinal tract may bleed, with consequent hematemesis, melena, severe iron-deficiency anemia and even death.

LABORATORY FINDINGS

Iron-deficiency anemia is common in blue rubber-bleb nevus syndrome. X-rays may reveal many polypoid filling defects throughout the length of the bowel. These defects may also be visualized easily by fiberoptic endoscopy. Computed tomography scans and magnetic resonance imaging often help to determine the full extent of involvement by the angiomatosis.

HISTOPATHOLOGICAL FINDINGS

The features consist of very widely dilated vein-like structures in the dermis and the subcutaneous fat, some of which may thrombose and become organized (Fig 19.3), and of cavern-like hemangiomas together with some changes of angiokeratoma that affect the lamina propria and submucosa in the gastrointestinal tract.

51

ETIOLOGY AND PATHOGENESIS

The cause of blue rubber-bleb nevus syndrome is a mutation in the gene situated in the chromosome 9p.

MANAGEMENT

Cutaneous lesions that are particularly troublesome may be excised surgically. Laser therapy has been used to provide excellent results in removal of the vascular nevi. Hemorrhage from the gastrointestinal tract may be controlled endoscopically.

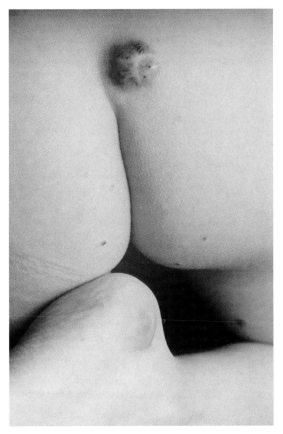

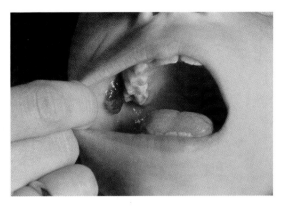

Figure 19.2
Blue rubber-bleb nevus syndrome. The nodule on the buccal mucosa is benign because is well circumscribed and symmetrical. It has a mahogany hue and it glistens.

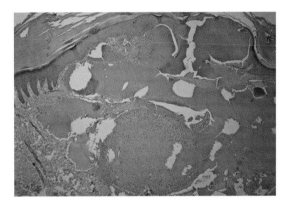

Figure 19.1
Blue rubber-bleb nevus syndrome. There are several papules and nodules. The nodule above and to the right of the intergluteal fold is gray–black. The nodule behind the malleolus is slightly bluish. Such a lesion is easily herniated by gentle pressure and is not painful to pressure.

Figure 19.3
Blue rubber-bleb nevus syndrome. With scanning magnification, a striking vascular malformation can be seen extending from the subcutaneous fat to immediately beneath the thinned epidermis.

20 BROMODERMA

Bromoderma is a skin eruption caused by ingestion of bromides. It is similar to eruptions caused by other halogens such as iodides and fluorides.

EPIDEMIOLOGY

Bromoderma is now rare in children. It has no predilection for any race or for either sex.

CLINICAL FINDINGS

The clinical lesions of bromoderma vary with the stage of the disease. The earliest lesions are often papules that quickly become pustular and resemble those seen in acne vulgaris. As the process evolves, vesicles and bullae tend to form, which may leave large residual ulcers when they rupture. The ulcers often develop crusts in their centers (Fig. 20.1) and pustules along their peripheries.

Vegetations are seen mainly in adolescents as reddish-blue, heaped-up crusts that are most prominent on the lower legs (Fig. 20.2). The mucous membranes, hair and nails are not usually affected. The lesions persist unless exposure to halogens is terminated.

LABORATORY FINDINGS

Blood levels of halogens may be elevated, but levels do not correlate with the severity of the disease. The total leukocyte count is often raised, and extremely high eosinophilia (68%) has been noted.

HISTOPATHOLOGICAL FINDINGS

The inflammatory process of bromoderma primarily affects hair follicles (Figs 20.3 and 20.4). The affected follicles are characterized by marked dilatation of the infundibula, which are filled with neutrophils, and by infundibular hyperplasia that sometimes is so striking as to be 'pseudocarcinomatous'. Prominent scaly crusts are present on the surfaces of some lesions. A dense, mixed inflammatory cell infiltrate (composed mostly of neutrophils, but also of lymphocytes and histiocytes) is present in the upper part of the dermis.

ETIOLOGY AND PATHOGENESIS

The exact manner in which halogens induce the eruptions is not known.

MANAGEMENT

The offending halogen must be withdrawn. Compresses followed by powerful topical corticosteroids are adjuncts to termination of the halogen.

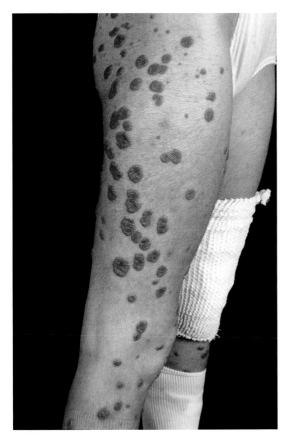

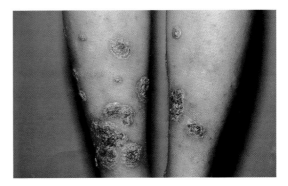

Figure 20.2
Bromoderma. Many plaques are covered by vegetations and are surrounded by rims of dusky erythema. The vegetations consist of both scales and crusts.

Figures 20.3 and 20.4
Bromoderma. This papillated lesion is characterized by widely dilated follicular infundibula plugged by ortho-keratotic and parakeratotic cells and filled by abscesses. Polymorphonuclear leukocytes are present, mostly within hyperplastic follicular infundibula but also within the dermis and within the scaly crusts.

Figure 20.1
Bromoderma. There are many roundish papules and plaques, and the borders of the plaques are partially elevated. At this stage the lesions consist mostly of hemorrhagic and purulent crusts.

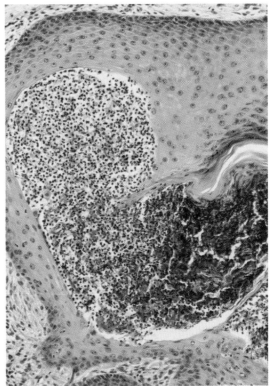

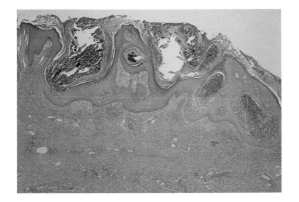

Figure 20.3

Figure 20.4

BULLOUS PEMPHIGOID

Bullous pemphigoid is a blistering disorder characterized by tense subepidermal vesicles and bullae.

EPIDEMIOLOGY

Bullous pemphigoid is rare in children. The onset is usually in the first decade of life.

CLINICAL FINDINGS

The disease presents first as urticarial papules and plaques and then as tense, discrete vesicles and bullae (Figs 21.1 and 21.2). The blisters cannot be extended centrifugally by pressing against their edges (Nikolsky's sign). Furthermore, urticarial plaques do not always result in blisters. The lesions of bullous pemphigoid usually affect the flexural areas and the lower part of the abdomen. Erosions in the mouth secondary to rupture of blisters are rare but are more frequent in children than in adults with the disease. The erosions in the oral cavity may be painful. At times, cutaneous bullae are hemorrhagic.

LABORATORY FINDINGS

Direct immunofluorescence reveals deposits in linear array of immunoglobulin G at the basement membrane zone in nearly all patients (Fig. 21.3). Indirect immunofluorescence reveals circulating immunoglobulin G antibodies directed against basement membrane zone in about 70% of patients who have active disease.

HISTOPATHOLOGICAL FINDINGS

Urticarial lesions are characterized by a superficial perivascular and interstitial infiltrate of lymphocytes and eosinophils. Numerous eosinophils are present within the upper part of the edematous dermis, and some of them may even be present in the epidermis, where spongiosis of variable extent is seen. The blister that develops in the lamina lucida is subepidermal and contains eosinophils (Fig. 21.4). Papillae at the base of the blister are usually preserved.

ETIOLOGY AND PATHOGENESIS

The source of the autoantibodies that are thought to be responsible for the disease is unknown.

MANAGEMENT

The agents of choice for treating bullous pemphigoid in children are systemic corticosteroids. Prednisone (1–2 mg/kg per day) almost always controls the disease. The dose should be tapered and discontinued as quickly as possible. Dapsone is an effective adjuvant, which may exert an effect that permits less use of corticosteroids.

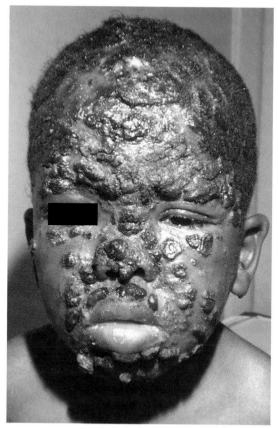

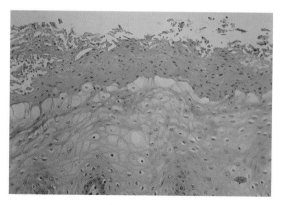

Figure 22.6

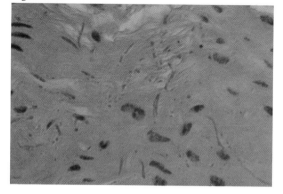

Figure 22.7

Figure 22.5
Chronic mucocutaneous candidiasis. This extensive granulo-matous infection (candidal granuloma syndrome) results in markedly hyperkeratotic areas on the face of this immunocompromised child.

Figures 22.6 and 22.7
Candidiasis. Within the markedly thickened parakeratotic cornified layer are numerous pseudohyphae of *Candida albicans.*

23 CAT-SCRATCH DISEASE

Cat-scratch disease produces a primary lesion in the skin and a secondary regional lympadenopathy. It affects children and adults who have been scratched by a cat.

EPIDEMIOLOGY

Cat-scratch disease is mostly a disease of the young and is worldwide in distribution. The disease usually occurs after the age of 3 years, when children begin to play with pets. The skin lesions appear 3–10 days after the scratch of a cat.

CLINICAL FINDINGS

The initial lesion, appearing 3–10 days after a cat scratch at the site of a scratch, is a red papule, 5–10 mm in diameter, which may ulcerate and become covered by a crust (Fig. 23.1). The lesion is usually situated on the limbs or face. Regional lymph node enlargement, without signs of lymphangitis, is noticeable 3–12 weeks after the appearance of the primary lesion and is characterized by red, painful and tender lymph nodes (Fig. 23.2). Nodes suppurate and become confluent in about 20% of patients. Low-grade fever, headache, anorexia, nausea, malaise, myalgia and arthralgia are seen in about a one-third of patients. The primary lesion persists for about 1–2 months. Regional lymphadenopthy usually regresses after a few weeks.

LABORATORY FINDINGS

A positive skin test with Hanger–Rose antigen (induration of more than 5 mm after 72 hours) is indicative of cat-scratch disease.

HISTOPATHOLOGICAL FINDINGS

Confirmation of the diagnosis may be obtained by demonstration of the causative agent with the Warthin–Starry silver stain.

ETIOLOGY AND PATHOGENESIS

The cause of cat-scratch disease is a Gram-negative organism, *Bartonella hanselae*.

MANAGEMENT

Cat-scratch disease subsides without therapy. Incision and drainage of affected lymph nodes should be avoided because fistulas may develop. The efficacy of therapy with tetracyclines and other antimicrobial agents remains controversial.

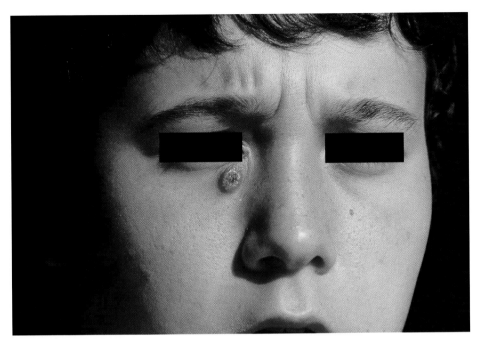

Figure 23.1
Cat-scratch disease. This relatively well-circumscribed, reddish-brown nodule is centrally ulcerated and covered by crusts.

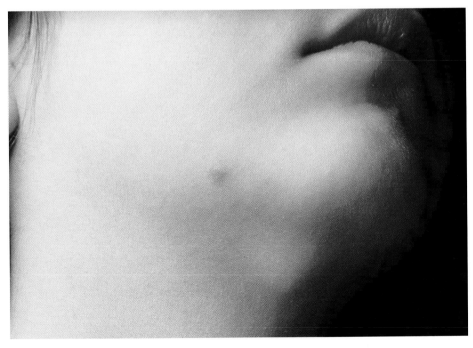

Figure 23.2
Cat-scratch disease. Below and to the left of the small, pink, smooth-surfaced papule is a substantial swelling that represents an enlarged lymph node.

24

CHEILITIS

CHEILITIS GLANDULARIS

Cheilitis glandularis is characterized by a prominent lower lip. It is caused by hyperplasia of the salivary glands and ducts.

EPIDEMIOLOGY

Cheilitis glandularis is an extremely rare disorder observed as early as the first decade of life.

CLINICAL FINDINGS

Cheilitis glandularis consists of painless enlargement and eversion of the lower lip caused by hyperplasia of the salivary glands and ducts. The involved lip has a cobbled surface (Fig. 24.1), and patulous openings of the salivary ducts are visible easily on its surface. Mucus can be extruded from the openings by squeezing the firm lip gently. It has a chronic course.

Complications

Rarely, intense suppuration leads to abscesses, fistulous tracts, ulcers and purulent crusts. This form of the disease has also been called cheilitis glandularis apostematosa. The most serious complication is the development of squamous cell carcinomas.

HISTOPATHOLOGICAL FINDINGS

The salivary glands are enlarged. The salivary ducts within the substance of the glands, the lamina propria and the surface epithelium are widely dilated by abundant acid mucopolysaccharide (mucin). Sometimes, rupture of the distended ducts results in discharge of the mucin into the lamina propria. In response to extravasated mucin, a variably dense patchy infiltrate of inflammatory cells forms. It is suppurative initially; later it is composed mostly of lymphocytes and histiocytes.

ETIOLOGY AND PATHOGENESIS

The cause of cheilitis glandularis is not known.

MANAGEMENT

No treatment for cheilitis glandularis has been successful. Wedge resections of the inner aspect of the lip or vermilionectomy are used to correct cosmetic disfigurement that results from the swollen lip

CHEILITIS GRANULOMATOSA

Cheilitis granulomatosa is characterized by swelling of the lips caused by granulomatous inflammation.

EPIDEMIOLOGY

Cheilitis granulomatosa is an extremely rare disorder. The vast majority of patients are girls.

CLINICAL FEATURES

Cheilitis granulomatosa is characterized by episodes of swelling of the lips that ultimately lead to persistently enlarged lips (Fig 24.2). This sign is one feature of Melkersson–Rosenthal syndrome, which consists of facial swelling, paralysis of a facial nerve and plicate tongue. The swelling is not accompanied by erythema, pruritus or tenderness. The acute episodes last for days only but with each recurrence, the swelling persists longer and becomes progressively more firm. The lips are often everted, which causes the moist surface of mucous membranes to be exposed to air. This results in chapping and fissuring.

HISTOPATHOLOGICAL FINDINGS

The lesions are characterized by granulomas composed of epithelioid histiocytes and surrounded by lymphocytes and plasma cells within the dermis, the subcutaneous fat and skeletal muscle (Figs 24.3 and 24.4).

ETIOLOGY AND PATHOGENESIS

The cause of cheilitis granulomatosa is not known.

MANAGEMENT

There is no satisfactory treatment for cheilitis granulomatosa. Facial swelling may be decreased by corticosteroids injected into the zone of involvement at about monthly intervals. The cosmetic deformity caused by protruding lips may be ameliorated somewhat by wedge resection of the inner margin of the lips. Intralesional injections of corticosteroids should be maintained after surgery to diminish the chances of recurrence.

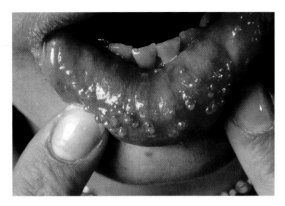

Figure 24.1
Cheilitis glandularis. When the lower lip is folded, as shown here, many glistening translucent papules are revealed. Such papules are full of acid mucopolysaccharides.

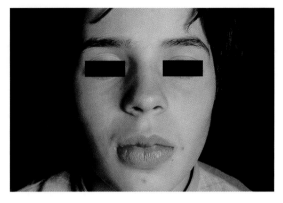

Figure 24.2
Cheilitis granulomatosa. The lower lip of this adolescent is markedly swollen as a consequence of granulomatous involvement of the tissues.

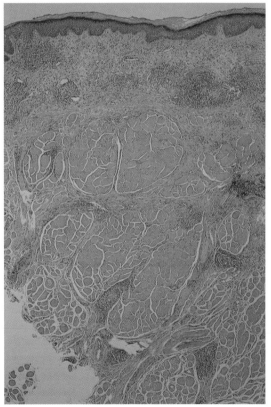

Figure 24.3

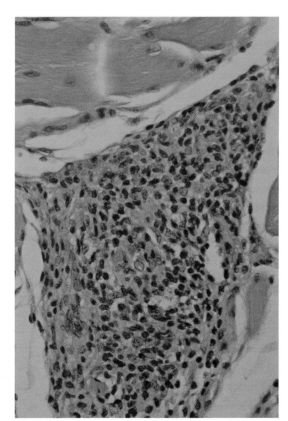

Figure 24.4

Figures 24.3 and 24.4
Cheilitis granulomatosa. Collections of epithelioid histiocytes surrounded by lymphocytes in the lamina propria, submucosa and skeletal muscle of the lip.

25

CONGENITAL MELANOCYTIC NEVI

Congenital melanocytic nevi are proliferations of melanocytes present at birth, or very soon after birth, in the skin and sometimes in the tissues beneath it.

EPIDEMIOLOGY

Congenital melanocytic nevi are present in almost 1% of white newborns.

CLINICAL FINDINGS

Congenital nevi vary considerably in size, shape, color, surface characteristics, and degree of hairiness. Congenital nevi are conventionally subdivided into small (from less than 15 mm up to 50 mm in greatest diameter to) (Fig. 25.1), large (50–200 mm) (Figs 25.2 and 25.3), and giant (greater than 200 mm) (Fig. 25.4).

The color varies from light brown to dark brown or black. Small congenital nevi are usually oval or round; large or giant congenital nevi may assume irregular shapes. The borders may be sharply demarcated or they may merge imperceptibly with surrounding skin.

Congenital nevi may have an uneven 'pebbled cobblestone' and rough surface with or without long coarse and dark hairs. The consistency is usually soft or wormy.

Associations

Large congenital nevi situated in the area of the head and neck may be associated with leptomeningeal melanocytosis and attendant neurological findings, including seizures. Similarly, large congenital nevi in the lumbosacral area may be associated with defects in the underlying spinal column such as meningomyelocele or spina bifida.

Complications

The single most important complication within a congenital nevus is development of malignant melanoma. A giant congenital nevus has a 10–20% chance of having a malignant melanoma develop within it, whereas a small congenital nevus has a less than 1% chance of being the harbinger of a malignant melanoma.

HISTOPATHOLOGICAL FINDINGS

In small congenital nevi, melanocytes are splayed between collagen bundles in the reticular dermis and there is angiocentricity and adnexocentricity of melanocytes (Figs 25.5 and 25.6). Large congenital nevi consist of dense diffuse infiltrate of melanocytes throughout the dermis and often in the subcutaneous fat. Giant congenital nevi may also contain melanocytes below the subcutis; melanocytes may be seen in large blood vessels such as veins in the septa of subcutaneous fat.

ETIOLOGY AND PATHOGENESIS

The cause of congenital nevi is not known, but genetic factors are surely important. They are presumed to occur as a result of a developmental defect in neural crest-derived melanocytes.

MANAGEMENT

Considerable debate continues, without resolution, about the management of both small and large congenital nevi. Many authors contend that all congenital nevi, irrespective of size, should be excised at puberty, when local anesthesia is possible. In giant congenital nevi the risk of melanoma is significant even in the first 3–5 years of life and therefore this type of nevus should be removed as soon as possible. Tissue expanders and tissue cultures using the patient's own normal skin can be used to facilitate removal of very large lesions.

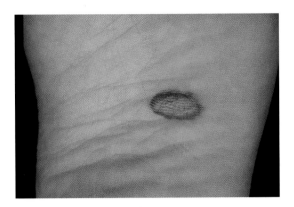

Figure 25.1
Small congenital nevus. This lesion, on the sole, is benign because it is symmetrical in shape, uniform in coloration and relatively well circumscribed.

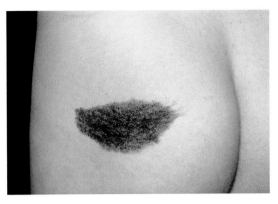

Figure 25.2
Large congenital nevus. This lesion consists of many dark brown papules situated on a tannish patch. Numerous fine hairs cover the nevus.

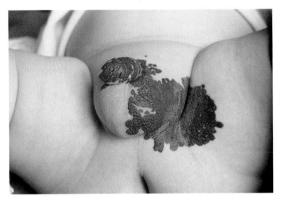

Figure 25.3
Large congenital nevus. This bizarre-shaped, uniformly colored bluish-black plaque has a scalloped and reticulated periphery that, nonetheless, is sharply circumscribed – a sign that it is benign.

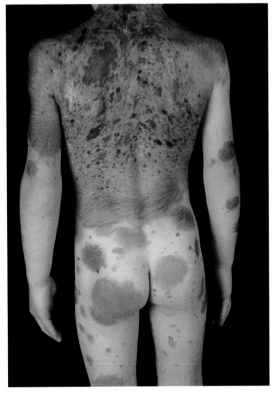

Figure 25.4
Giant congenital nevus. All the widespread pigmented lesions in this boy are congenital nevi. Some are hairy, others are not. Some of the lesions on the shoulders and back are difficult to differentiate clinically from malignant melanomas.

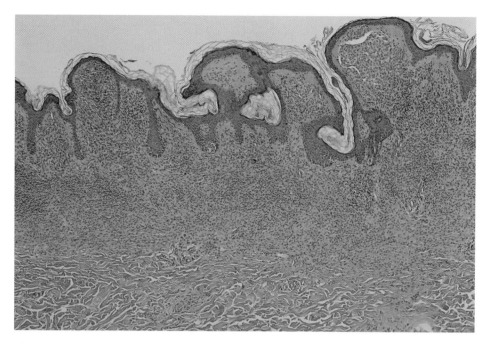

Figure 25.5

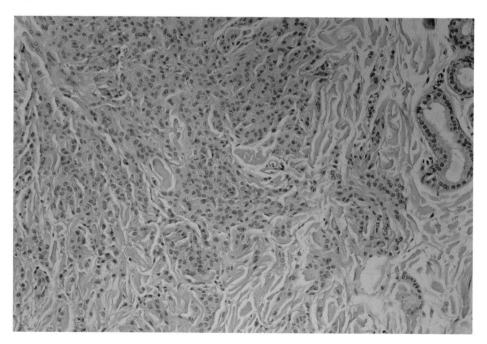

Figure 25.6

Figures 25.5 and 25.6

Small congenital nevus. This nevus is characterized by involvement of the upper half of the dermis and by sparing of the lower half. The melanocytes of the reticular dermis are arranged in two distinct patterns – around blood vessels and between collagen bundles.

26

CONNECTIVE TISSUE NEVI

Connective tissue nevi are malformations characterized by excessive amounts of either collagen or elastic tissue and sometimes of mucin.

EPIDEMIOLOGY

Connective tissue nevi are rare disorders, although their incidence is probably underestimated.

CLINICAL FINDINGS

Collagenous nevi

Connective tissue nevi that are marked by an excess of collagen are called collagenous nevi or collagenomas. They may be congenital or acquired, solitary or multiple. The lesions consist of asymptomatic yellow–brown or skin-colored patches, papules, nodules or plaques of variable sizes and shapes (Figs 26.1 and 26.2). Their mammillated surfaces have often been compared to that of pigskin. They are usually situated on the trunk or the extremities and persist for life.

Four subtypes of collagenomas have been described:

- isolated collagenoma (Fig. 26.1), which is a patch or plaque in zosteriform distribution that is not associated with other diseases;
- eruptive collagenoma (Fig. 26.2), which presents suddenly with numerous macules that quickly become papules and then nodules;
- familial cutaneous collagenoma, which is typified by numerous, symmetrically

distributed nodules and is often associated with extracutaneous abnormalities, particularly cardiac problems;
- Shagreen patch (better termed 'plaque' because its mammillated surface is raised above the surface of surrounding normal skin), which occurs in the lumbosacral area of children with tuberous sclerosis.

Elastic tissue nevi

Connective tissue nevi marked by an excess of elastic tissue are called elastic tissue nevi or elastomas. They, like collagenomas, may be congenital or acquired, solitary or multiple. The commonest forms taken by these hamartomas are:

- dermatofibrosis lenticularis disseminata, which consists of numerous elastic tissue nevi in association with osteopoikilosis (mesenchymal alterations of bone). Taken together, these findings constitute the Buschke–Ollendorff syndrome. The cutaneous lesions are small, asymptomatic papules distributed symmetrically on the lower part of the trunk or the extremities;
- Solitary elastoma, which is a plaque composed of yellowish papules (nevus elasticus of Lewandowsky) or nodules (juvenile elastoma) and is situated principally on the trunk and buttocks; it is seemingly without genetic transmission (Fig. 26.3).

HISTOPATHOLOGICAL FINDINGS

Connective tissue nevi are characterized by alteration in quality and quantity of collagen and elastic tissue in the absence of associated inflammation or neoplasia. Collagenous nevi have thickened collagen bundles, some of which are oriented vertically to the skin surface. The reticular dermis may be thickened (Fig. 26.4). Elastic tissue nevi usually have markedly thickened fibers, either focally or diffusely, within the reticular dermis.

Etiology and Pathogenesis

The accumulation of collagen and elastin seems to result primarily from overproduction of these substances at a molecular level. A precise molecular defect has yet to be defined.

Management

Collagenous and elastic tissue nevi in themselves are harmless and rarely need to be removed except for cosmetic considerations. The simplest and most effective way to remove them is surgical excision.

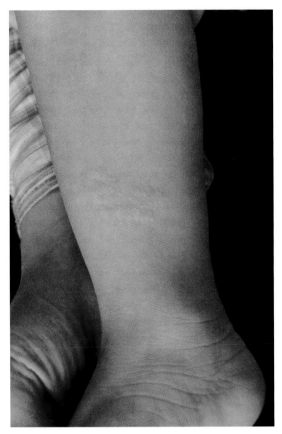

Figure 26.1
Isolated collagenoma. The skin-colored plaque is ill-defined and characterized by a slightly mamillated surface.

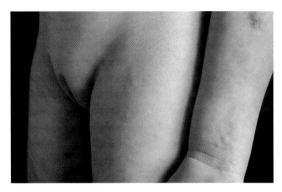

Figure 26.2
Eruptive collagenoma. There are papules and plaques of 'collagenoma' along the left forearm and thigh. The lesions have a smooth surface and are of skin-colored, tan or reddish-brown hues.

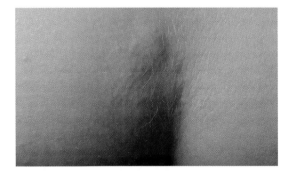

Figure 26.3
Solitary elastoma. Skin colored papules have become confluent to form a slightly elevated plaque.

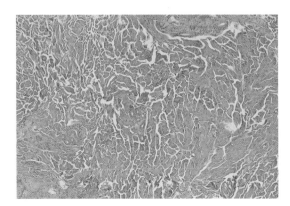

Figure 26.4
Collagenous nevus. Dense collagen bundles arranged mostly horizontally but also vertically to the skin surface thicken the dermis of this mamillated lesion of shagreen plaque.

27

CONTACT DERMATITIS

Contact dermatitis is an inflammatory reaction. It either occurs within several days of direct contact with an allergen (allergic contact dermatitis) or follows immediately after direct contact with an irritant (irritant contact dermatitis).

EPIDEMIOLOGY

Allergic contact dermatitis occurs in only a small percentage of children who have been exposed to the sensitizing agent. Irritant contact dermatitis is very common in infants.

CLINICAL FINDINGS

Allergic contact dermatitis follows re-exposure to a sensitizing agent and requires several days between first exposure and the development of the dermatitis. In the acute phase the dermatitis consists of well-demarcated plaques of erythema and edema on which vesicles exuding serum and crusts are superimposed (Figs 27.1 and 27.2). In the subacute phase the erythematous plaques show papules and desquamation. The chronic phase consists of plaques of lichenification (thickening of epidermis with enhanced skin lines) and signs of excoriations. All the objective signs are accompanied by itching. The distribution and shape of the lesions depend on the nature of the allergen and often provide clues to its detection. 'Id' reactions (i.e. development of lesions similar to those at the primary site of allergic contact dermatitis, but distant from it) are not uncommon.

Irritant contact dermatitis occurs quickly after first exposure to an irritant. It is charac-

terized by well-defined plaques of erythema, vesicles, blisters and erosions (Fig. 27.3). Irritant contact dermatitis usually bypasses the papular stage and, in the subacute stage, crusts and scaling predominate. The commonest example of irritant contact dermatitis in young children is diaper (nappy) dermatitis.

HISTOPATHOLOGICAL FINDINGS

Early lesions of allergic contact dermatitis are characterized by superficial perivascular and interstitial infiltrates composed mostly of lymphocytes (but sometimes of variable numbers of eosinophils), edema of the papillary dermis, and focal spongiosis that may eventually result in spongiotic vesicles (Fig. 27.4).

Fully developed lesions show a somewhat denser infiltrate of similar composition, more marked edema of dermal papillae, psoriasiform hyperplasia, spongiotic vesicles, and scaly crusts composed of parakeratosis and plasma.

Late lesions are marked by features of lichen simplex chronicus, a consequence of vigorous and prolonged rubbing of the persistent pruritic lesions of allergic contact dermatitis. The findings are of compact orthokeratosis, hypergranulosis, irregular psoriasiform hyperplasia and a papillary dermis thickened by coarse collagen bundles that are oriented perpendicular to the skin surface and parallel to the rete ridges.

Irritant contact dermatitis is characterized by superficial perivascular and interstitial infiltrates of lymphocytes and neutrophils, ballooning of epidermal keratinocytes, ballooning vesiculation and necrosis of keratinocytes.

LABORATORY FINDINGS

Patch tests are necessary to prove a sensitization. In children who are younger than 5 years of age, concentration of the agents used in patch tests should be adjusted (usually to one-half of adult concentration).

ETIOLOGY AND PATHOGENESIS

In children, the most frequent causes of allergic contact dermatitis are nickel (in jewellery), dichromates (in shoes), phenylenediamine, balsam of Peru, neomycin, sulfonamides, antihistamine creams, and rubber in shoes. Among cosmetics, agents that most commonly cause allergic contact dermatitis are moisturizing and cleansing agents, antiperspirants, lipsticks and eye make-up, in that order. The commonest allergenic ingredients in cosmetics are fragrances, followed by preservatives (such as Kathon CG or parabens) and emulsifiers. In the first year of life, allergic contact dermatitis is nearly always a consequence of topically applied vioform, neomycin, or penicillin. Allergic contact dermatitis is an example of type IV delayed hypersensitivity.

Irritant contact dermatitis differs from allergic contact dermatitis because it is not immunologically mediated.

MANAGEMENT

The agent responsible for allergic contact dermatitis should be sought vigorously. Irritants are usually easier to recognize than allergens by history and physical examination. Treatment consists of elimination of the causative allergen or irritant. This alone should bring relief, albeit slowly. Prompt improvement can be effected by topical application of corticosteroids. If there is severe oozing and crusting, compresses with plain water or agents such as aluminium hydroxide should be applied before topical corticosteroids are brought in contact with the affected site. Systemic corticosteroids may be indicated in rare circumstance. Antihistamines help to diminish pruritus, but have no other benefits.

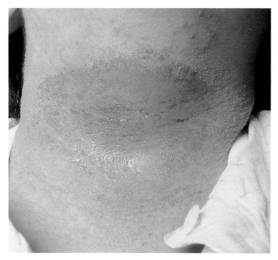

Figure 27.1
Allergic contact dermatitis. Scales, crusted papules and vesicles provide a rim around a weeping erosion. The cause of this dermatitis was topically applied neomycin.

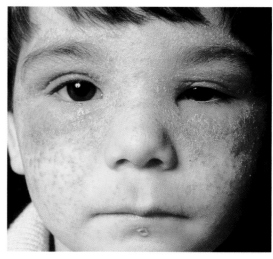

Figure 27.2
Allergic contact dermatitis. In addition to prominent edema of periorbital skin bilaterally, there are papules covered by gray scales and yellow crusts. The dermatitis was a consequence of eyedrops that contained an antibiotic.

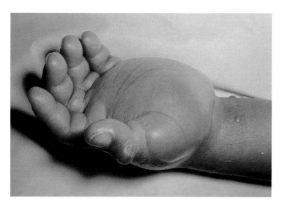

Figure 27.3
Irritant contact dermatitis. The vesicles and bullae were caused by an irritant in this child's mitten. The blisters developed quickly (hours) after the mitten was first worn.

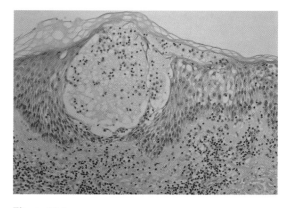

Figure 27.4
Allergic contact dermatitis. This is an early lesion because there is only a single discrete spongiotic vesicle despite the several zones of spongiosis. Furthermore, the cornified layer has a basket-weave configuration devoid of parakeratosis or scaly crusts, a sign of a lesion that is only a few days old.

DARIER'S DISEASE

Darier's disease is a genodermatosis that is characterized clinically by rough, gray–brown, mostly non-follicular papules that are localized predominantly on the face and the upper part of the trunk. Histopathologically it is characterized by foci of acantholytic and dyskeratotic cells.

EPIDEMIOLOGY

Darier's disease is uncommon but not rare.

CLINICAL FINDINGS

The fundamental lesions of Darier's disease are brownish keratotic papules (Figs 30.1 and 30.2), which may become confluent to form plaques. Sites of predilection are the 'seborrheic areas,' which include the face, the preauricular areas and the ears, the neck, the chest and the midline of the back. Commonly, flat wart-like papules are present on the dorsa of the hands and the feet. Punctate keratoses, either raised or with a central pit, may be seen on the palms and soles. The nails are commonly affected in Darier's disease, and increased brittleness, longitudinal splits and V-shaped notches of the distal part of the nail plate are typical findings. Lesions tend to appear from the age of 5 years through to adolescence. The disease is persistent and long-standing. It is exacerbated during summer and after exposure to ultraviolet light. The oral mucosa in patients with Darier's disease may be affected by white papules clustered in a 'cobblestone' pattern.

Complications

Patients with Darier's disease are susceptible to widespread cutaneous infections by viruses such as herpes simplex, vaccinia and Coxsackie viruses. Less frequently, bacteria or fungi may infect the lesions of Darier's disease.

HISTOPATHOLOGICAL FINDINGS

Darier's disease is characterized by foci of suprabasal clefts, acantholytic dyskeratotic cells in the spinous and granular layers (Figs 30.3 and 30.4) and columns of parakeratotic cells, some of which are acantholytic

ETIOLOGY AND PATHOGENESIS

Darier's disease is inherited as an autosomal-dominant trait. The site of altered gene has been localized in 12q23–24.1

MANAGEMENT

'Keratolytic' ointments and creams that contain all-trans retinoic acid are beneficial. Some children with Darier's disease benefit from oral retinoids, but others do not. Treatment with either 13-cis-retinoic acid or etretinate should be started at a low dose of 0.5 mg/kg per day in two divided doses and increased gradually if needed.

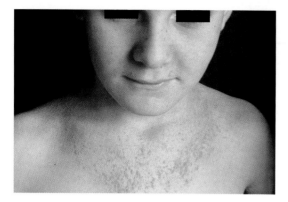

Figure 30.1
Darier's disease. Red–brown keratotic papules are present in semilunar configuration on the upper part of the chest, where they are confined to sites exposed to sunlight.

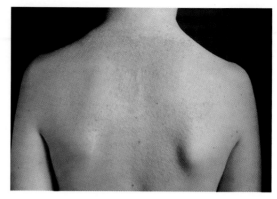

Figure 30.2
Darier's disease. Red–brown keratotic papules are present in somewhat wedge-shaped distribution on the back.

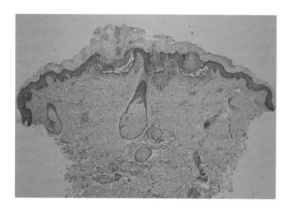

Figure 30.3

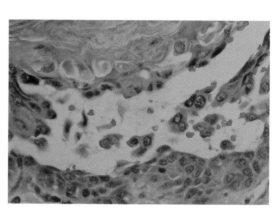

Figure 30.4

Figures 30.3 and 30.4
Darier's disease. Several foci of acantholytic dyskeratosis are apparent within the epidermis. Each focus is characterized by a suprabasal cleft, above which acantholytic dyskeratotic cells are present in the spinous, granular and cornified layers. Each focus is topped by column of parakeratosis.

31 DERMATITIS HERPETIFORMIS

Dermatitis herpetiformis is a chronic disorder associated with gluten enteropathy. It is characterized clinically by intensely pruritic papules and vesicles that tend to be grouped in herpetiform fashion. Histopathologically it is characterized by subepidermal vesicles in dermal papillae, in which there are numerous neutrophils.

EPIDEMIOLOGY

The prevalence varies from one person per 10,000 to one person per 80,000, depending on the population studied. In children the peak age of onset is between 3 and 6 years.

CLINICAL FINDINGS

Dermatitis herpetiformis is typified by pink, edematous (urticarial) papules and by vesicles distributed symmetrically over the shoulders, especially the scapulae, the elbows, the back, the sacrum, the buttocks and the knees (Figs 31.1, 31.2, 31.3 and 31.4). Herpetiform grouping of lesions is a helpful, but inconstant, diagnostic feature. Sometimes the only signs are crusted erosions or ulcerations, which are the result of vigorous excoriation, or post-inflammatory hypopigmentation (see Figs 31.1 and 31.4). A child with dermatitis herpetiformis may complain of stinging, burning or itching of the skin, any one of which may herald eruption of fresh papules and vesicles. Ingestion of iodides or overload of gluten dramatically exacerbates the eruption. In the absence of specific therapy, lesions of dermatitis herpetiformis can persist into adulthood.

Associations

A gluten-dependent enteropathy, characterized by patchy atrophy of jejunal villi, occurs in nearly all patients. Immunoglobulin A antibodies binding to the intermyofibril substance of smooth muscle (antiendomysial antibodies) are present in the majority of patients. The incidence of HLA-B8 and DR3 is markedly increased compared with the general population.

LABORATORY FINDINGS

Direct immunofluorescence reveals granular deposits of immunoglobulin A, as well as deposits of complement (C3) and fibrin, at the tips of dermal papillae in the skin around the lesions (Fig. 31.8). Circulating basement membrane zone antibodies are generally not detectable in the serum of patients, although immunocomplexes have been found in 20–40% of patients.

HISTOPATHOLOGICAL FINDINGS

The papules are characterized by collections of neutrophils, neutrophilic nuclear dust, a variable number of eosinophils, microabscesses in dermal papillae (Figs 31.5 and 31.6) and by subepidermal clefts that may contain fibrin. Vesicles are subepidermal and contain mostly neutrophils but also eosinophils (Fig. 31.7).

ETIOLOGY AND PATHOGENESIS

The presence of granular deposits of immunoglobulin A at the dermoepidermal junction and the association of dermatitis herpetiformis with gluten-sensitive enteropathy indicate that a defective mucosal immune response may be pivotal to the development of this disorder in genetically predisposed people. However, the relationship of the gluten-sensitive enteropathy to the skin lesions has been controversial. Following loading of gluten by ingestion, patients develop increased levels of circulating immune complexes to gluten–immunoglobulin A, which are deposited in dermal papillae. Subsequent activation of complement, chemotaxis of neutrophils and release of neutrophilic mediators lead to tissue injury.

MANAGEMENT

In most children, cutaneous and intestinal manifestations of dermatitis herpetiformis may be controlled within 1–6 months of starting a gluten-free diet. Although all types of cutaneous lesions of dermatitis herpetiformis respond dramatically to therapy with dapsone, the accompanying intestinal disorder is unaffected by dapsone. In patients who are unresponsive to diet alone, a combination of gluten restriction and dapsone therapy enables the daily dose of dapsone to be reduced markedly. Patients taking dapsone must have their glucose-6-phosphate dehydrogenase level measured before and during therapy, because dapsone may induce catastrophic hemolysis in patients who are deficient in this enzyme.

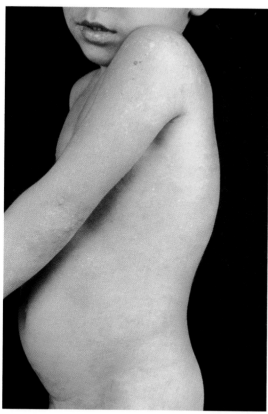

Figure 31.1
Dermatitis herpetiformis. Urticarial papules and crusts are situated near the elbows, and foci of post-inflammatory hypopigmentation are present on the shoulders. Some of the papules have become confluent to form small plaques.

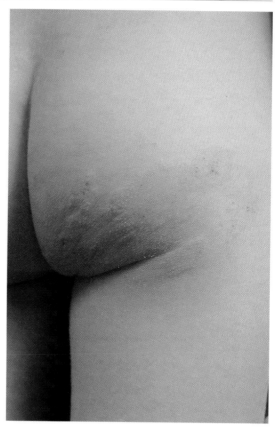

Figure 31.3
Dermatitis herpetiformis. On the buttocks of this child a plaque made up of an edematous papule and vesicles is evident.

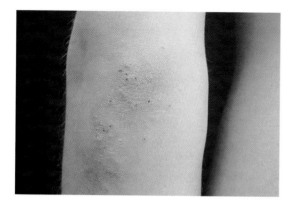

Figure 31.2
Dermatitis herpetiformis. Herpetiform grouping of lesions is a typical diagnostic feature.

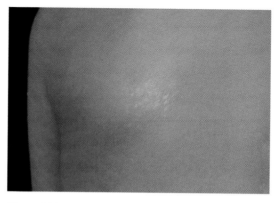

Figure 31.4
Dermatitis herpetiformis. The characteristic distribution of the hypopigmented macule is virtually diagnostic of this disease.

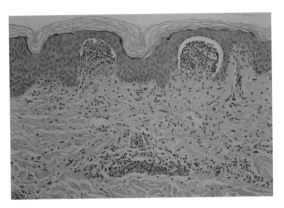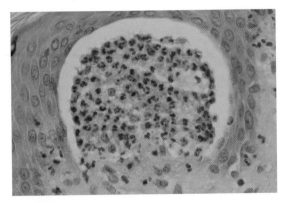

Figure 31.5

Figure 31.6

Figures 31.5 and 31.6
Dermatitis herpetiformis. Numerous neutrophils are positioned in subepidermal spaces and dermal papillae.

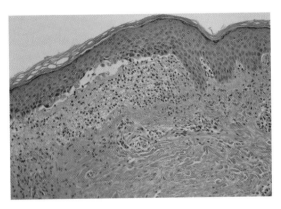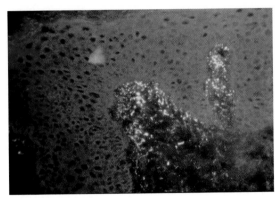

Figure 31.7
Dermatitis herpetiformis. A subepidermal blister contains neutrophils and eosinophils.

Figure 31.8
Dermatitis herpetiformis. Direct immunofluorescence. Most granules of immunoglobulin A are situated near the top of dermal papillae.

DERMATOFIBROMA

EPIDEMIOLOGY

Dermatofibroma is the commonest fibro-histiocytic proliferation in adults but it is rare in children.

CLINICAL FINDINGS

Dermatofibromas (Fig. 32.1) are well-defined, usually asymptomatic papules and nodules that range in size from a few millimeters to more than 20 mm, with a mean of about 10 mm. They have a predilection for the extremities, especially the legs. Their color ranges from pink to dark brown and tends to vary from the center of the lesion to the edge. Dermatofibromas, on palpation, can be appreciated to be much deeper lesions than they appear to be on inspection; only a small portion of their mass is elevated above the surface of the skin. Over the course of many years, however, dermatofibromas become progressively flatter and may eventually become depressed below the surface of the surrounding skin.

HISTOPATHOLOGICAL FINDINGS

Dermatofibromas consist of a proliferation of histiocytes and fibrocytes within the dermis, with thickened bundles of collagen at the periphery of the lesion (Fig. 32.2). There is epidermal hyperplasia with hyperpigmentation.

ETIOLOGY AND PATHOGENESIS

In general, dermatofibromas appear within weeks or months after an injury, often a penetrating one.

MANAGEMENT

Dermatofibromas are best left alone. They flatten in time. Surgical excision may be employed for cosmetic purposes. Cryosurgery has been claimed to be effective in some patients.

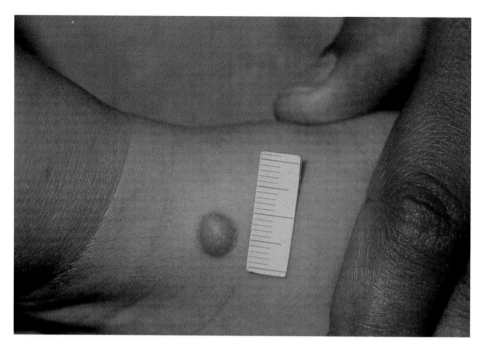

Figure 32.1
Dermatofibroma. This dome-shaped, red–brown, firm nodule appeared a few weeks after a
penetrating trauma.

Figure 32.2
Dermatofibroma. Numerous fibrocytes and histiocytes are seen to be associated with coarse bundles
of collagen. All the components are arrayed haphazardly.

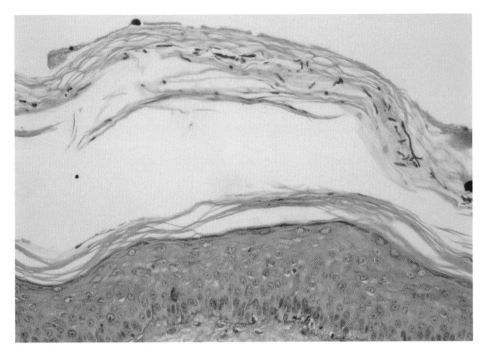

Figure 35.7
Dermatophytosis. The thickened cornified layer is seen teeming with hyphae.

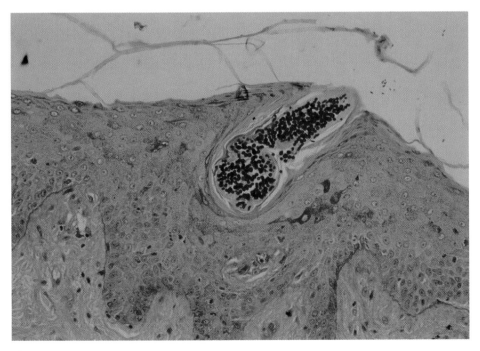

Figure 35.8
Dermatophytosis. The hair shaft and the inner sheath are both filled with fungi.

DIAPER DERMATITIS

'Diaper dermatitis,' also known as 'nappy dermatitis,' is an inflammatory condition that occurs in infants and that follows the combined effects of occlusion and irritation in the diaper region.

EPIDEMIOLOGY

This condition was very common in Europe and North America in the 1970s but it is now much rarer owing to improvements in the quality of disposable diapers.

CLINICAL FINDINGS

Clinically, diaper dermatitis is typified at first by shiny, reddish macules that tend to become confluent and form plaques (Fig. 36.1). Lesions are usually limited to convex surfaces of the pubic region, the genitalia, the buttocks, and the upper part of the thighs. At times, discrete, barely elevated, flat-topped, oval papules may accompany the plaques. In long-lasting cases, papules or nodules, which may be isolated or grouped and fully evolved or ulcerated, may be present. These are known as syphiloid dermatitis of Sevestre–Jacquet (Fig. 36.2). In other cases, one or more red–brown nodules and tumors, measuring as much as several centimeters in diameter, arise on convex areas as well as in the crural region. These large, dark nodular and tumorous lesions have been termed granuloma gluteale infantum (Fig. 36.3). Without treatment, diaper dermatitis is likely to persist until the use of diapers stops.

Complications

Secondary infection of diaper dermatitis by staphylococci and *Candida albicans* is frequent.

HISTOPATHOLOGICAL FINDINGS

Fully developed lesions of diaper dermatitis (i.e. granuloma gluteale infantum) are slightly domed and characterized by compact orthokeratosis, marked hypergranulosis, irregular psoriasiform or pseudocarcinomatous hyperplasia, prominent edema of the upper part of the dermis, and a dense, usually patchy infiltrate, made up predominantly of neutrophils, in the upper half of the dermis. The infiltrate is not monomorphous, however, but contains numerous lymphocytes and plasma cells in addition to neutrophils (Figs. 36.4 and 36.5). Karyophagocytosis is common.

ETIOLOGY AND PATHOGENESIS

Many factors are thought to play a causative role in diaper dermatitis. Among them are friction caused by paper or plastic diapers, excessive humidity and maceration, prolonged contact with urine and feces, ammonia produced by the breakdown of urea, secondary bacterial infections, irritation by chemicals contained in diapers or used in cleaning them, and irritation by soap and detergents. However, there is as yet no evidence that links any of these factors conclusively and definitively to the causation of diaper dermatitis.

MANAGEMENT

The frequency of diaper dermatitis correlates directly with the duration of skin contact with feces, and inversely with how often nappies are changed. Therefore, nappies should be changed as often as possible if diaper dermatitis is to be avoided. Tight-fitting diapers also should be avoided and plastic diapers should be shunned entirely. The skin should not be washed with soap but with warm water only. Every effort must be made to keep the skin dry. Non-infectious inflammatory changes may be managed with such time-tested preparations as zinc oxide cream or Lassar's paste. In the Sevestre–Jacquet form of the condition, topical preparations of antibiotics may be used for a few days to decrease likelihood of bacterial infection through erosions. Occlusive agents and potentially irritating agents should not be used.

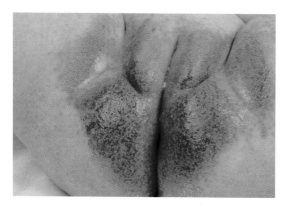

Figure 36.1
Diaper dermatitis. These bright red plaques are eroded, crusted and scaly. Many tiny papules are seen at their periphery.

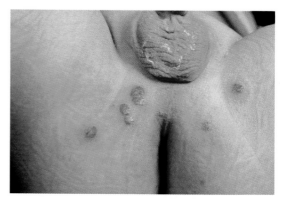

Figure 36.2
Diaper dermatitis. Syphiloid dermatitis of Sevestre–Jacquet. The red–brown papules and nodules covered by scaly crusts resemble lesions of secondary syphilis. The changes are but one manifestation of diaper dermatitis

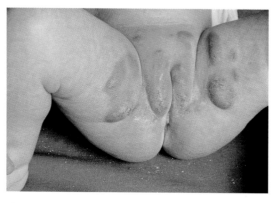

Figure 36.3
Granuloma gluteale infantum. Numerous papules and nodules are situated on top of the plaques. The brown hue indicates that the lesions are long standing. Crusts and scaly crusts cover the erosions and ulcerations.

Figures 36.4 and 36.5
Granuloma gluteale infantum. The lesion is domed because of a dense, brown patchy, lichenoid infiltrate of inflammatory cells. In the upper part of the dermis, blood vessels are dilated. The pallor is evidence of edema. Neutrophils are present within the hyperplastic epidermis. In other foci, lymphocytes and plasma cells predominate.

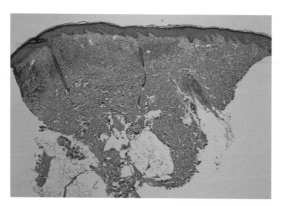

Figure 36.4

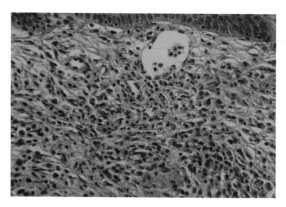

Figure 36.5

37

DYSHIDROTIC DERMATITIS

Dyshidrotic dermatitis, known also as pompholyx and dyshidrosis, is an inflammatory disease in which papules and vesicles are situated mostly on the palms and the soles and along the sides of the fingers and toes.

EPIDEMIOLOGY

Dyshidrotic dermatitis is uncommon before 10 years of age and exceptional before 5 years. From the second decade of life onwards, dyshidrotic dermatitis is among the commoner inflammatory diseases of the skin.

CLINICAL FINDINGS

Tense vesicles, which tend to become coalescent to resemble tapioca, arise along the sides of the fingers. They may ultimately involve an entire palm (or sole) or both (Figs 37.1 and 37.2). If vesicles become confluent, bullae may result. Itching is variable but is often severe. Dyshidrotic dermatitis has an unpredictable course, waxing and waning without apparent cause.

Complications

Extensive vesiculation and secondary infections may cause serious disability by compromising the function of the hands and feet.

HISTOPATHOLOGICAL FINDINGS

Foci of spongiosis and spongiotic vesicles, edema of the papillary dermis, and a superficial, perivascular, predominantly lymphocytic infiltrate are findings in evolving lesions of dyshidrotic dermatitis (Fig. 37.3).

ETIOLOGY AND PATHOGENESIS

The cause of dyshidrotic dermatitis is not known. Despite the name there is no evidence that excessive sweating plays a role. The disease occurs more often in patients with atopic dermatitis. Emotional stress is a possible precipitating factor.

MANAGEMENT

No treatment is consistently effective for dyshidrotic dermatitis, although many have been advocated. Topical corticosteroids are widely used.

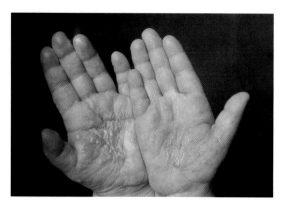

Figure 37.1
Dyshidrotic dermatitis. Nearly the entire volar surface is covered by tiny papules and vesicles, some of which have become confluent and others pustular. Near the wrists the confluence of tiny tense vesicles has eventuated in a multiloculated bulla that looks like tapioca.

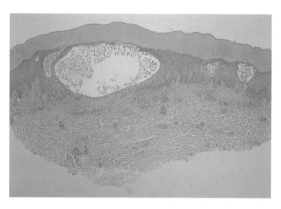

Figure 37.3
Dyshidrotic dermatitis. The lesion on volar skin is characterized by spongiosis and spongiotic vesiculation, psoriasiform hyperplasia and a superficial and mid-dermal (predominantly lymphocytic) infiltrate.

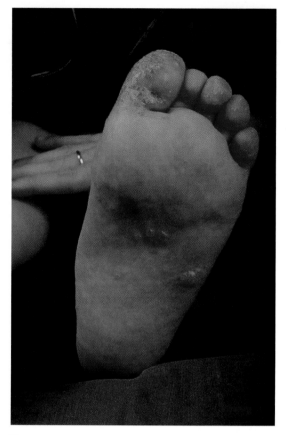

Figure 37.2
Dyshidrotic dermatitis. The toes and the plantar surface of the feet are affected by the inflammatory process at different stages of its evolution, from tiny vesicles to blisters.

Dyskeratosis congenita (Zinsser–Cole–Engman syndrome) is a rare genetic disorder characterized by a constellation of reticulated hyperpigmentation of the skin, dystrophy of the nails and leukokeratosis on mucous membranes.

EPIDEMIOLOGY

Dyskeratosis congenita is rare. It mainly affects males, and dermatological manifestations generally become evident before puberty.

CLINICAL FINDINGS

Dyskeratosis congenita usually presents itself as slowly progressive skin lesions in the form of reticulate, lacy hyperpigmentation (Fig. 38.1) sometimes accompanied by interspersed zones of hypopigmentation.

Nail dystrophy is found in 98% of patients with dyskeratosis congenita and is expressed as longitudinal grooves in the nails, thinned nails or nearly complete atrophy of the nails.

Leukokeratosis (Fig. 38.2) is present in about 85% of patients and tends to appear on the buccal and lingual mucosa.

Other dermatological manifestations include palmoplantar hyperhidrosis (in 87% of patients), bullae (in 78%), epiphora – a persistent overflow of tears caused by obstruction of the lachrymal ducts and often one of the first symptoms (in 78%), hyperkeratosis of the palms and soles (in 72%), taurodont teeth (in 63%) and aberrations of hair, including alopecia (in 51%).

Hematologic abnormalities occur in more than half of the patients and, as a rule, manifest themselves some time in the second decade of life. Failure of bone marrow to function, with subsequent pancytopenia, is common, as are aplastic anemia, bleeding, and recurrent infections.

Increased susceptibility to neoplasia is characteristic in nearly half of the patients. The neoplasms usually become apparent by the third decade of life. They tend to affect mucous membranes (squamous cell carcinoma in areas of leukoplakia), the pancreas (adenocarcinoma) and the lymph nodes (Hodgkin's disease).

LABORATORY FINDINGS

Anemia is present in about half of patients and is usually the first expression of cytopenia. Neutropenia and thrombocytopenia usually follow shortly, although they may not appear for many years after the onset of anemia. Myeloid and erythroid progenitors in bone marrow are reduced or absent.

HISTOPATHOLOGICAL FINDINGS

The epidermis is thinned focally and is devoid of rete ridges in the thinned foci. Vacuolar alteration is found beneath zones of thinned epidermis. Melanophages and a sparse perivascular infiltrate of lymphocytes are often present in the upper part of the dermis (Figs 38.3 and 38.4). On mucous membranes there may be marked orthokeratosis and parakeratosis, slightly elongated but broadened rete ridges, and variable degrees of nuclear atypia of keratinocytes within the broadened rete ridges.

ETIOLOGY AND PATHOGENESIS

Dyskeratosis congenita is inherited in X-linked fashion, and the responsible gene has been assigned to the Xq 28 locus.

MANAGEMENT

No effective therapy for dyskeratosis congenita is known. Patients with the syndrome should be kept under close observation to detect early signs of bone marrow failure and malignant neoplasms. Topical retinoids may help to decrease leukokeratosis.

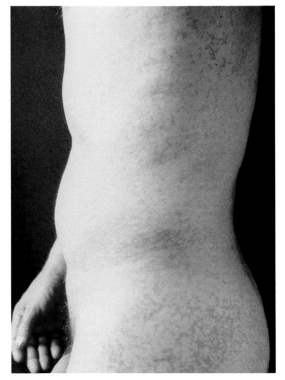

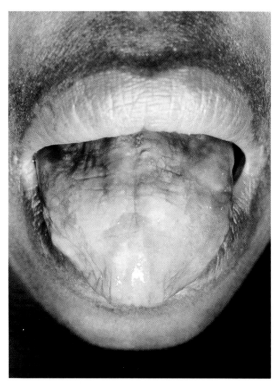

Figure 38.1
Dyskeratosis congenita. Reticulated hyperpigmentation in a patchy distribution covers much of the trunk, the flank and the buttocks of this adolescent.

Figure 38.2
Dyskeratosis congenita. White plaques on the tongue of this black adolescent are a consequence of hyperkertosis. The changes could represent an early stage in the evolution of squamous cell carcinoma.

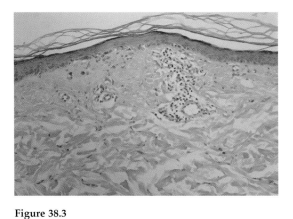

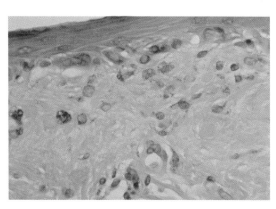

Figure 38.3

Figure 38.4

Figures 38.3 and 38.4
Dyskeratosis congenita. There is a sparse, perivascular, lymphocyte infiltrate beneath a thinned epidermis. The infiltrate obscures the dermoepidermal junction focally, where vacuolar alterations can be seen. Melanophages are present in the upper part of the dermis.

39   EHLERS–DANLOS SYNDROME

Ehlers–Danlos syndrome is not a true syndrome, but a group of at least 10 different disorders characterized by systemic aberration of connective tissue. Hyperelastic or friable skin and hypermobile joints are the findings that most of these disorders have in common.

EPIDEMIOLOGY

Ehlers–Danlos syndrome as a whole is uncommon but not rare.

CLINICAL FINDINGS

The skin in Ehlers–Danlos syndrome is soft, velvety and extremely elastic (Fig. 39.1). In children, once the altered skin has been stretched and released, it returns immediately to its normal position. Increased fragility of the skin in those afflicted by Ehlers–Danlos syndrome causes the skin to split in response to even minor trauma, with resultant formation of atrophic scars of different sizes and shapes (Fig. 39.2). The scars are most commonly situated over bony prominences and extensor surfaces of joints. Healing is slow and sutures repeatedly fail to hold. Areas of trauma also may be sites for development of soft 'molluscoid pseudotumors', which represent abnormal accumulations of collagenous and adipose tissue. The skin bruises easily and hematomas form frequently. Hyperextensibility of joints (Figs 39.3 and 39.4) may result in dislocations, kyphoscoliosis, genu recurvatum and hallux valgus. Hyperextensibility may be so extreme that walking

becomes difficult. Varicose veins may develop in children with the syndrome. Ten forms of Ehlers–Danlos syndrome have been described to date (Table 39.1), and these differ in clinical manifestations, mode of inheritance, and underlying pathological defect. The disease may not become clinically apparent until the child begins to crawl or even to walk. In the absence of visceral involvement, patients may have a normal life span.

ETIOLOGY AND PATHOGENESIS

The causes of Ehlers–Danlos syndrome are described in Table 39.1.

HISTOPATHOLOGICAL FINDINGS

As a rule, conventional microscopy reveals no abnormalities in the skin of patients with Ehlers–Danlos syndrome.

MANAGEMENT

Genetic counselling is crucial to women with types I or IV Ehlers–Danlos syndrome because of the risk of premature rupture of membranes and because of maternal morbidity and mortality. Avoidance of trauma and the use of pressure dressings after trauma are helpful in preventing both cutaneous and joint complications. A surgeon should be highly alert to a diagnosis of Ehlers–Danlos syndrome before performing any operation because of difficulties inherent in the healing of wounds.

Table 39.1 Clinical features, mode of inheritance, and biochemical defect in Ehlers–Danlos syndrome

Type	Main clinical feature	Inheritance	Biochemical defect
I (Gravis)	Hyperextensible, velvety skin; easy bruising; atrophic scars; hypermobile joints; prematurity	Autosomal dominant	Unknown
II (Mitis)	As in type I, but less severe	Autosomal dominant	Unknown
III (Benign hypermobile)	Marked joint hypermobility; skin manifestations almost absent	Autosomal dominant	Unknown
IV (Ecchymotic)	Thin and translucent skin; little joint hypermobility; arterial manifestations; rupture of bowel sometimes	Autosomal dominant or autosomal recessive	Abnormal type III collagen
V (X-linked)	Similar to type II	X-linked	Unknown
VI (Ocular)	Hyperextensible, velvety skin; hypermobile joints; scleral and corneal fragility (recessive)	Autosomal recessive	Lysyl hydroxylase deficiency
VII (Arthrocholasis)	Multiple dislocations; joint hypermobility; soft multiplex skin; scars not abnormal	Autosomal dominant or autosomal recessive	Procollagen conversion abnormality
VIII (Periodontal)	Generalized periodontitis; skin and joint mobility similar to type II	Autosomal dominant	Unknown
IX (Cutis laxa and occipital horn)	Lax, extensible skin; bladder diverticula; inguinal hernias; skeletal abnormalities (recessive)	X-linked	Abnormal copper utilization with deficiency of lysyl oxidase
X (Fibronectin defect)	Similar to type II	Autosomal recessive	Fibronectin defect

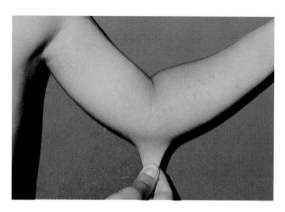

Figure 39.1
Ehlers–Danlos syndrome. Even a gentle tug on the skin elicits dramatic hyperextensibility.

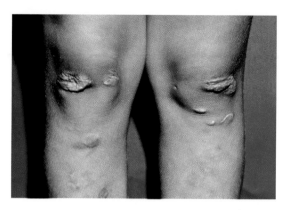

Figure 39.2
Ehlers–Danlos syndrome. There are numerous atrophic scars, like those of anetodermas at sites of previous traumas. Because this condition is characterized by fragility of the skin, subtle trauma may induce scars like these.

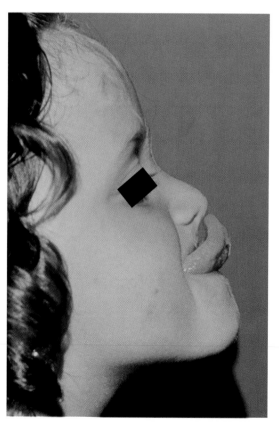

Figure 39.3
Ehlers–Danlos syndrome. Some patients can touch their noses with the tip of their tongues. Note also the atrophic hypopigmented scar on the forehead.

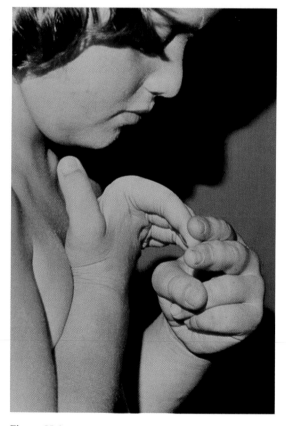

Figure 39.4
Ehlers–Danlos syndrome. This child demonstrates remarkable hyperextensibility of her joints.

ELASTOSIS PERFORANS SERPIGINOSA

Elastosis perforans serpiginosa consists of papules, usually in annular or arcuate configurations. The papules are characterized histopathologically by channels within the surface epithelium; these channels contain altered elastic fibers.

EPIDEMIOLOGY

The disease is uncommon; in about 40% of patients it begins between ages 5 and 10 years.

CLINICAL FINDINGS

The papules of elastosis perforans serpiginosa are asymptomatic, skin-colored to red and keratotic (Fig. 40.1) or crusted. Some of the papules may be umbilicated. Typically, they are 2–5 mm in diameter and are arranged in arcuate (Fig. 40.2), annular and serpiginous patterns. Sites of predilection are the posterolateral aspects of the neck, the arms, the elbows, the knees and the antecubital fossae. Lesions improve without treatment within 5–10 years.

Associations

About 30% of patients with elastosis perforans serpiginosa also are afflicted by one or more other genodermatoses, such as Ehlers–Danlos syndrome, Marfan's syndrome or pseudoxanthoma elasticum. The disease is especially frequent in people with Down's syndrome.

HISTOPATHOLOGICAL FINDINGS

Elastosis perforans serpiginosa is characterized by an increase in the number of thickened, highly eosinophilic, elastic fibers in the upper part of the dermis and within channels that extend through the surface epithelium, where neutrophils and neutrophilic debris also are lodged (Figs 40.3 and 40.4).

ETIOLOGY AND PATHOGENESIS

Except in the case of lesions induced by penicillamine, the cause of elastosis perforans serpiginosa is not known.

MANAGEMENT

Treatment of elastosis perforans serpiginosa is generally unsatisfactory. Favorable results have been described with liquid nitrogen and stripping with cellophane tape, but only in a few patients.

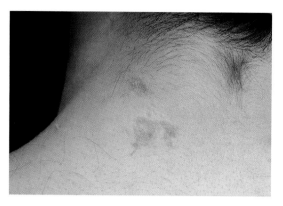

Figure 40.1

Elastosis perforans serpiginosa. Numerous reddish papules with a slight violaceous hue have become confluent to form a small plaque. Scrutiny of the papules reveals a subtle dell within them.

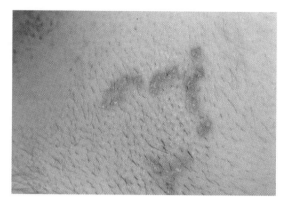

Figure 40.2

Elastosis perforans serpiginosa. The rust-colored keratotic papules situated near the base of the hairline on the posteriolateral neck are arranged in an arcuate pattern rather than a serpiginous pattern.

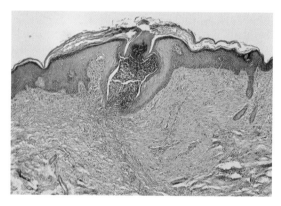

Figure 40.3

Figures 40.3 and 40.4

Elastosis perforans serpiginosa. The epithelial channels shown here are bounded by parakeratosis above and elastic fibers below. Within the channels are numerous neutrophils associated with thick elastic fibers, some of which are stained brightly eosinophilic; others are basophilic.

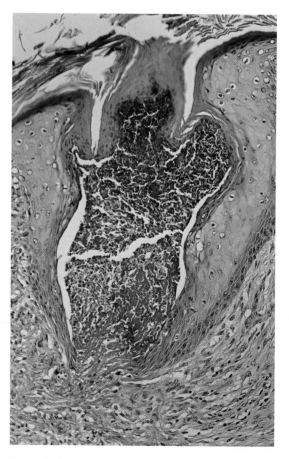

Figure 40.4

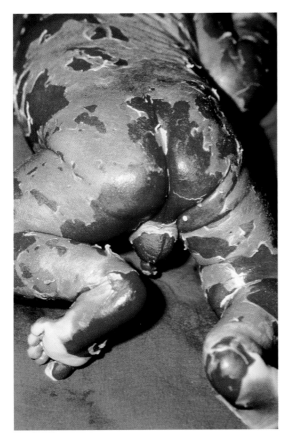

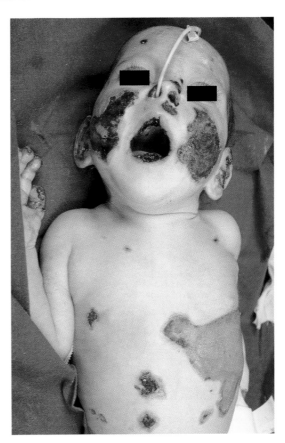

Figure 41.6

Junctional epidermolysis bullosa (Herlitz type). The whole skin of this infant is affected by large bullae that weep when they break, leaving erosions.

Figure 41.7

Junctional epidermolysis bullosa (Herlitz type). Severe recurring erosions are visible on the face and the trunk of this infant.

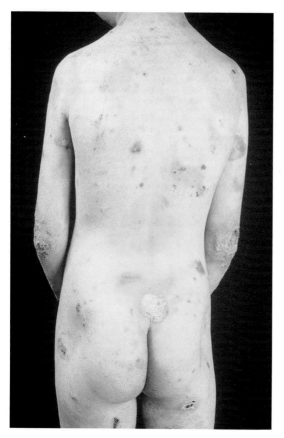

Figure 41.8
Junctional epidermolysis bullosa (non-Herlitz type). Widespread bullous lesions and atrophic scars are present both on trunk and limbs of this young girl.

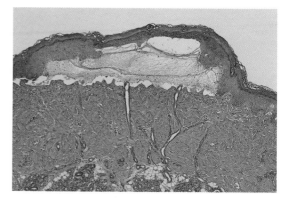

Figure 41.9
Junctional epidermolysis bullosa. A subepidermal blister is seen to contain fibrin but few inflammatory cells.

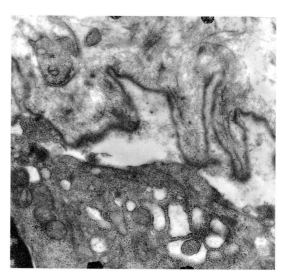

Figure 41.10
Junctional epidermolysis bullosa. By ultrastructure, blisters are located in the lamina lucida, and hypoplastic or rudimentary hemidesmosomes are characteristic.

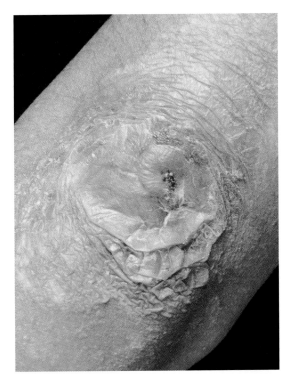

Figure 41.11
Dermolytic epidermolysis bullosa (widespread dominant dystrophic type). The extensive atrophic scars on an elbow are a consequence of recurrent subepidermal blisters at this site.

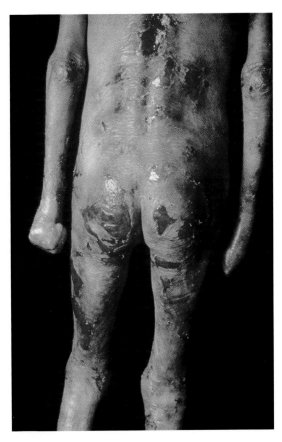

Figure 41.12
Dermolytic epidermolysis bullosa (recessive type). Widespread bullae and large ulcerations leave scars and cicatricial constrictions.

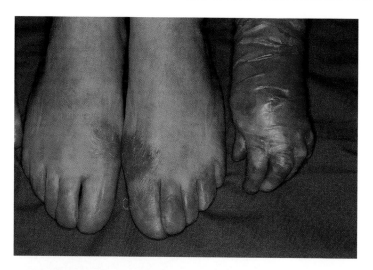

Figure 41.13
Dermolytic epidermolysis bullosa (recessive type). Frequent recurrence of blisters causes cicatricial fusion of the fingers and toes.

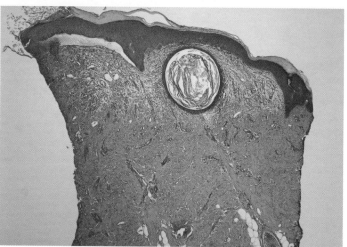

Figure 41.14
Dermolytic epidermolysis bullosa. A broad subepidermal blister extends along a folliculosebaceous unit.

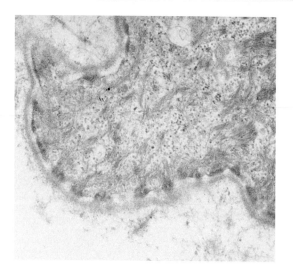

Figure 41.15
Dermolytic epidermolysis bullosa. Ultrastructural examination shows a blister below the lamina densa, with hypoplastic anchoring fibrils and normal hemidesmosomes.

EPIDERMOLYTIC HYPERKERATOSIS

Epidermolytic hyperkeratosis (also called bullous congenital icthyosiform erythroderma) is a widespread form of epidermal nevus.

EPIDEMIOLOGY

Epidermolytic hyperkeratosis is rare and is transmitted as an autosomal-dominant trait. However, many cases appear to be sporadic.

CLINICAL FINDINGS

Epidermolytic hyperkeratosis is usually present at birth. The affected newborn is erythrodermic and partially covered by large, flaccid bullae. As the bullae break, they leave residual weeping erosions. Erythroderma alone is seen early in the course and becomes less prominent after infancy, while blisters tend to develop only during the first year of life. After months or years, thick, malodorous gray–brown, verrucous keratotic lesions appear together with deep parallel furrows over virtually the whole skin surface. They are especially prominent on flexural surfaces of the extremities, which assume a rippled appearance (Figs 42.1 and 42.2). The hyperkeratotic lesions persist throughout life.

HISTOPATHOLOGICAL FINDINGS

Epidermolytic hyperkeratosis is characterized by a thickened epidermis in which the normal cohesive organization of spinous and granular cells has been replaced by a markedly vacuolated and feathery appearance, together with clumps of keratohyaline granules. The cornified layer is compactly orthokeratotic (Figs 42.3 and 42.4).

ETIOLOGY AND PATHOGENESIS

The most plausible explanation for epidermolytic hyperkeratosis is mosaicism (i.e. the presence within a single organism of two or more genetically distinct cell lines).

MANAGEMENT

Treatment is unsatisfactory. Oral retinoids may be useful for improving hyperkeratosis, but they may cause an increased tendency to blister.

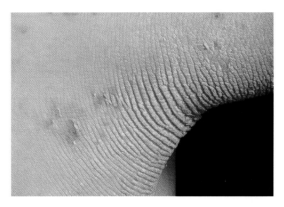

Figure 42.1

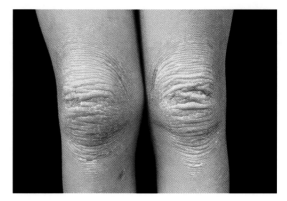

Figure 42.2

Figures 42.1 and 42.2
Epidermolytic hyperkeratosis. Keratotic papules arranged in parallel ridges and deep creases between these keratotic ridges give a rippled appearance to the flexures that is typical of this condition. The few erosions near the axillae presumably represent residua of blisters at that site.

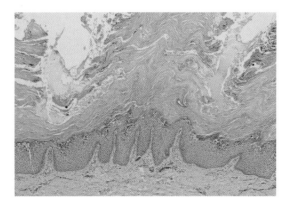

Figure 42.3

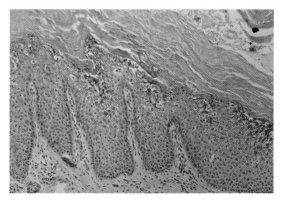

Figure 42.4

Figures 42.3 and 42.4
Epidermolytic hyperkeratosis. The cornified layer is approximately three times the thickness of the viable epidermis. Beneath prominent compact hyperkeratosis, the epidermis is seen to consist of a markedly increased number of kerato-hyaline granules, especially in its upper part, and of a feathery vacuolated appearance of keratinocytes in the spinous and granular zones. That feathery pattern is responsible for the misnomer 'epidermolytic'. In fact, there is no epidermolysis; the epidermal keratinocytes are cohesive.

43 ERYTHEMA ANNULARE CENTRIFUGUM

Erythema annulare centrifugum is an eruption of annular and arcuate red lesions that migrate slowly outwards. It is mainly seen in adults but it has been reported occasionally in children.

CLINICAL FINDINGS

Erythema annulare centrifugum consists of one or more lesions that begin as urticarial papules. The papules enlarge centrifugally to form polycyclic outlines that contain zones either of normal skin or of slightly hyperpigmented skin. The rims of the lesions may be firm, palpable and elevated (deep erythema annulae centrifugum) (Fig. 43.1) or erythematous with delicate scales on the inner position (superficial erythema annulare centrifugum) (Fig. 43.2). Sites of predilection are the trunk and upper limbs, but any part of the integument may be affected. Individual lesions tend to resolve within days or weeks, but new lesions continue to erupt. The condition may last for years. Although itching is present, it is absent in most patients.

HISTOPATHOLOGICAL FINDINGS

The two common types of erythema annulare centrifugum may be classified histopathologically as superficial or deep. The superficial type (Fig. 43.3) shows a superficial perivascular lymphocytic infiltrate, spongiosis in epidermal foci and mounds of parakeratosis. The deep type is characterized by a superficial and deep perivascular infiltrate of lymphocytes, without changes in the epidermis.

ETIOLOGY AND PATHOGENESIS

The causes of erythema annulare centrifugum remain obscure in the large majority of cases. Speculations about the cause in individual cases have included dermatophytes, viruses, infestations and drugs.

MANAGEMENT

Unless an underlying cause is found, no particular treatment has merit for this disease.

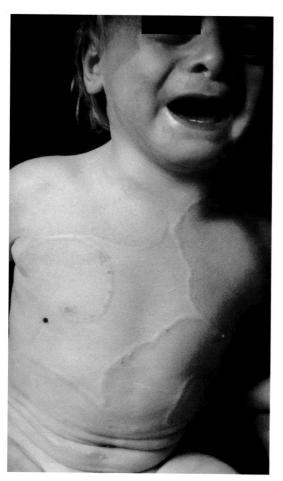

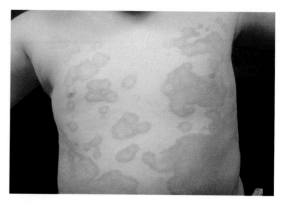

Figure 43.2

Erythema annulare centrifugum (superficial type). Widespread erythematous annular and polycyclic lesions with delicate scaling.

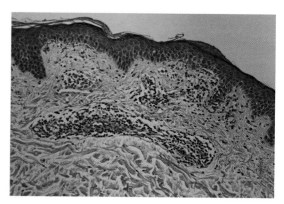

Figure 43.1

Erythema annulare centrifugum (deep type). Arcuate patterns are formed by urticarial lesions on the face and chest of this 4-year-old girl. The borders are sharply demarcated, smooth-surfaced and pink.

Figure 43.3

Erythema annulare centrifugum. Superficial perivascular lymphocytic infiltrate.

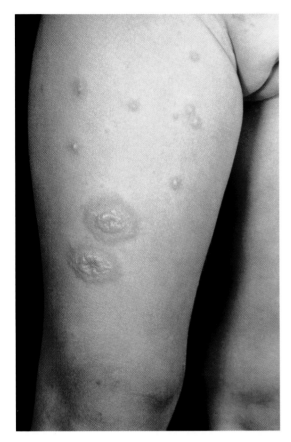

Figure 45.1
Erythema multiforme. The lesions may be papules, vesicles and blisters of different sizes. All three are present here. Concentric rings are characteristic of fully developed lesions.

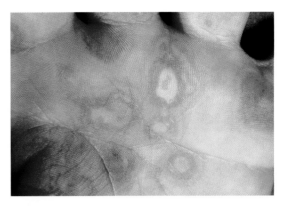

Figure 45.2
Erythema multiforme. The lesions tend to favor the acra, as here, and especially the palms and soles.

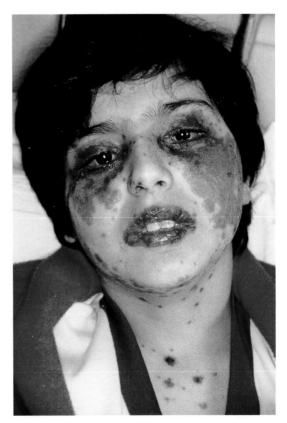

Figure 45.3
Erythema multiforme (Stevens–Johnson syndrome). The hemorrhagic papules and blisters have become confluent on the cheeks and around the eyes. Mucous membranes of the eyes, nose and mouth have been affected by the blistering process.

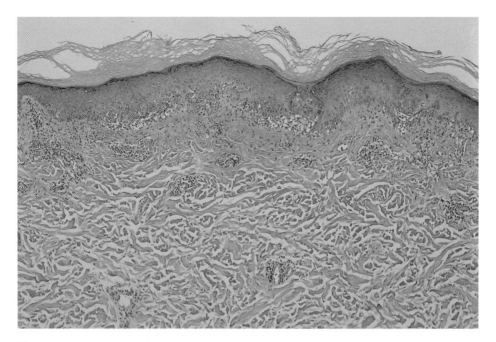

Figure 45.4

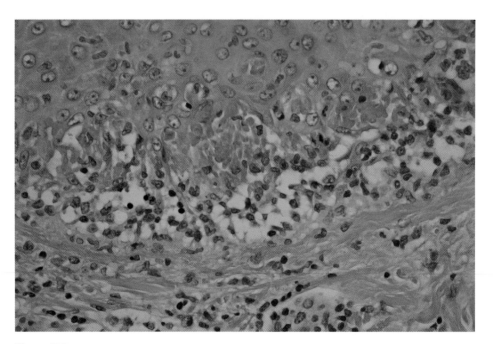

Figure 45.6

Figures 45.4 and 45.5

Erythema multiforme. Lymphocytes are present around vessels of the superficial plexus and along the dermoepidermal junction, where there is also vacuolar alteration. Note the spongiosis and ballooning and the numerous necrotic keratinocytes in the lower part of the epidermis.

Erythema nodosum is a distinctive panniculitis characterized by painful, red patches, plaques and nodules, which have a predeliction for the pretibial surfaces.

EPIDEMIOLOGY

Erythema nodosum is rare in the first 2 years of life. The peak incidence of this disease is the peripubertal period. Erythema nodosum is three times more common in females as in males.

CLINICAL FINDINGS

The onset of the lesions of erythema nodosum is often preceded by one or more symptoms and signs (fever, malaise, arthralgia, conjunctivitis or sore throat). Nodules (Figs 46.1 and 46.2) seem to develop rapidly and reach full size within 2 weeks. At first, the bright red, shiny lesions are macules or patches that range in diameter from less than 10 mm to more than 50 mm. These lesions soon become subtly raised, at which time they may be so exquisitely tender that even the weight of linen sheets may be unbearable and so painful that children may refuse to walk. Lesions are firm throughout their course. Their silhouettes tend to be round or oval, but their margins are poorly defined. Typically, only a few lesions are present, but 20 or more may be counted. The pretibial region is most frequently affected, followed by the upper part of the thighs and the buttocks. The lesions are bilateral, but not symmetrical. In most instances, about 10 days after the first lesion has appeared, no new lesions erupt. Within 3–6 weeks, nodules begin to resolve, the redness becomes progressively duller, and the lesions then acquire a purplish cast. As complete resolution nears, lesions take on a yellow–green hue that has prompted the appellation 'erythema contusiformis' because of the resemblance of late lesions of erythema nodosum to a fading bruise. Lesions of erythema nodosum do not suppurate, liquefy or ulcerate. Arthralgias are present in about 50% of patients and affect mainly the ankle joints. Although erythema nodosum is a self-limited disease, recurrences are frequent.

Associations

Erythema nodosum is known to occur in association with sarcoidosis, ulcerative colitis and Crohn's disease, Behçet's disease and erythema multiforme.

HISTOPATHOLOGICAL FINDINGS

In early lesions, scattered neutrophils are seen in slightly widened edematous septa in the subcutaneous fat.

Fully developed lesions are characterized by granulation tissue and granulomatous inflammation in markedly widened septa (Figs 46.3 and 46.4). Lobules affected by foam cells, fat microcysts and membranous fat necrosis appear to be constricted as a result of expansion of the septa.

In late lesions, fibrosing granulomatous inflammation and, eventually, fibrosis in markedly widened septa are observed.

ETIOLOGY AND PATHOGENESIS

Multiple and diverse etiologies have been proposed – tubercolosis, streptococcal infections, chlamydial infections, yersiniosis and histoplasmosis. In the majority of cases, no cause is identified. The precise pathogenesis of erythema nodosum, regardless of cause, also remains obscure.

MANAGEMENT

When the pain is disabling, salicylates and non-steroid anti-inflammatory drugs may be useful. The use of systemic corticosteroids is indicated only in severe cases after an infectious etiology has been excluded.

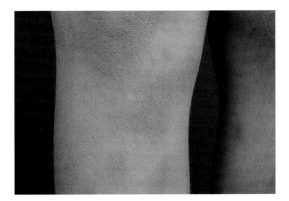

Figure 46.1
Erythema nodosum. The red nodules situated above the anterior tibia represent active evolving lesions of erythema nodosum.

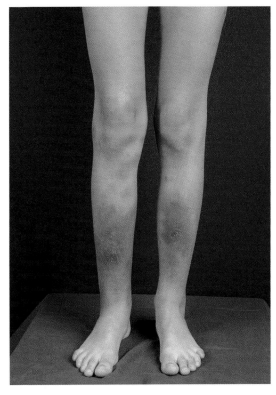

Figure 46.2
Erythema nodosum. The nodules are darkened and have become confluent to form plaques. These findings are expressions of late lesions of erythema nodosum.

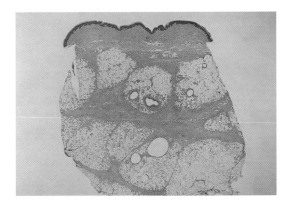

Figure 46.3

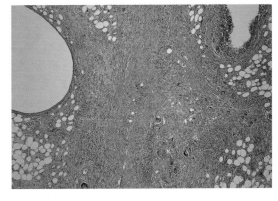

Figure 46.4

Figures 46.3 and 46.4
Erythema nodosum. At scanning magnification (Fig. 46.3), the subcutaneous fat is altered by widened septa that encroach on the fat lobules and constrict them. At higher magnification (Fig. 46.4), a granulomatous inflammation is evident.

47   ERYTHEMA TOXICUM NEONATORUM

Erythema toxicum neonatorum is a self-limited eruption peculiar to newborns. It is so prevalent that it can be considered normal. The condition is marked by widespread tiny pustules that usually occur between the 2nd and 4th days of life, but in many instances the onset may be at birth.

CLINICAL FINDINGS

Lesions usually begin as erythematous 'splotchy' macules (Figs 47.1 and 47.2) that may evolve into edematous papules. Although the lesions may remain macular or papular, many of them progress to tiny pustules. Individual lesions may coalesce, but they resolve without sequelae in a matter of days. The number of lesions ranges from very few to hundreds. Although the palms and soles are spared, the lesions can appear almost anywhere else, especially on the head and neck, the proximal parts of the extremities, the chest and the back.

HISTOPATHOLOGICAL FINDINGS

The lesions consist of collections of neutrophils and eosinophils in follicular infindibula.

ETIOLOGY AND PATHOGENESIS

The etiology and pathogenesis of erythema toxicum neonatorum remain mysterious, despite the commoness of the condition.

MANAGEMENT

No treatment is needed because the lesions are self-limited and disappear nearly as quickly as they develop.

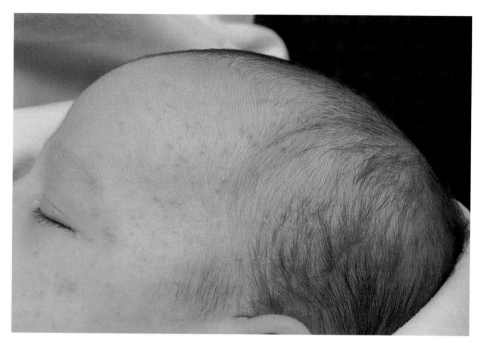

Figure 47.1
Erythema toxicum neonatorum. Discrete papules and papulopustules are scattered over the scalp and cheek of this newborn.

Figure 47.2
Erythema toxicum neonatorum. Macules, papules and tiny pustules are present on the dorsal and ventral surfaces of this newborn.

FIXED DRUG ERUPTION

Fixed drug eruption describes a distinctive cutaneous inflammatory process that is characterized clinically by a recurrence of circumscribed lesions in the same site or sites each time a particular offending drug or chemical is administered.

Epidemiology

The incidence of fixed drug eruption among children has been found to be 1 in 2000. The mean age at the time of onset is 7 years.

Clinical Findings

The earliest lesion of a fixed drug eruption is a well-defined, round or oval, red macule. This lesion occurs between 1 and 12 hours after ingestion of a drug in a previously sensitized person. Within a few days, the macule becomes a red–orange–violaceous plaque (Fig. 48.1) whose color closely resembles that of mercurochrome. A bulla may arise on the plaque. An original lesion is often solitary, but recurrent lesions tend to be multiple (Fig. 48.2). Recurrent lesions almost always appear at the exact site or sites of the original eruption. The extremities, the oral cavity, the perioral periorbital and perigenital areas, as well as the genitalia themselves, are the areas most commonly affected. Lesions may be confined to mucous membranes or they may be present on both the mucosae and the skin. Lesions rarely itch or burn. The lesions begin to regress within a few days once the offending drug has been withdrawn. They recur within hours after ingestion of the drug. With repeated attacks, lesions may increase in size and number, and the intensity of pigmentation and the likelihood of its persistence is increased.

Histopathological Findings

In early lesions a superficial and deep perivascular infiltrate that contains neutrophils and eosinophils obscures the dermoepidermal junction.

Fully developed lesions (Figs 48.3 and 48.4) are characterized by intraepidermal vesiculation secondary to vacuolar alteration and also by numerous necrotic keratinocytes within the epidermis and the upper part of epithelial structures of the adnexa.

In late lesions there are numerous melanophages within the papillary dermis.

Etiology and Pathogenesis

By definition, fixed drug eruption is induced by drugs. Tetracycline and phenolphthalein, sulfonamides and anti-inflammatory agents are the commonest precipitating drugs. The mechanisms of fixed drug eruption are not known.

Management

Identification and elimination of the drug responsible for the eruption is curative. Resolution of lesions may be hastened by the use of oral or topical corticosteroids.

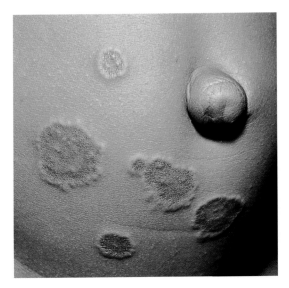

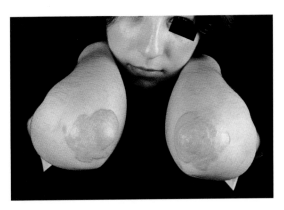

Figure 52.2
Granuloma annulare. There are red–brown, sharply demarcated plaques with discrete papules at the peripheries and within the centers on both elbows.

Figure 52.1
Granuloma annulare. These annular lesions are composed of numerous skin-colored papules. The brown contents represent post-inflammatory hyperpigmentation.

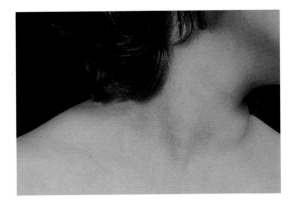

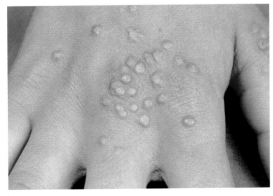

Figure 52.3
Granuloma annulare. This widespread form is manifested by tiny yellow–brown papules, some of which have a subtle annular configuration.

Figure 52.4
Granuloma annulare. Some of the discrete papules have a central dell that gives them an annular appearance. The slight scale on top of some of the papules is an unusual feature for conventional granuloma annulare but is expected for the perforating type.

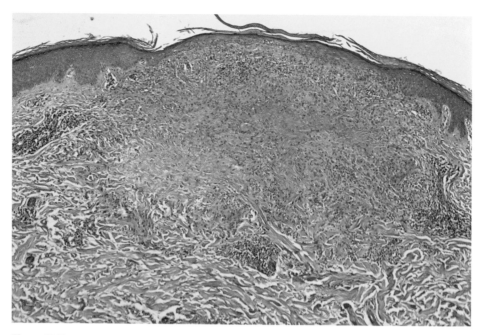

Figure 52.5

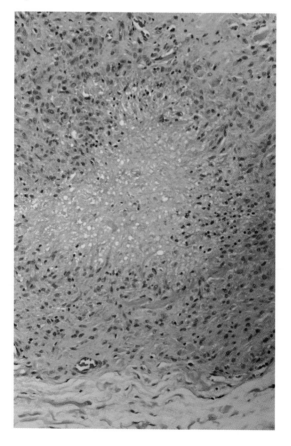

Figures 52.5. and 52.6
Granuloma annulare. Discrete foci of granulomatous inflammation are apparent through the reticular dermis. In each focus, histiocytes are seen to be aligned in a palisade around foci that contain abundant mucin and degenerated collagen.

Figure 52.6

53

HAND-FOOT-AND-MOUTH DISEASE

Hand-foot-and-mouth disease, usually caused by Coxsackievirus, is characterized clinically by an eruption of oblong or oval vesicles rimmed by redness on the distal part of the extremities and on the oral mucosa. Histopathologically it is characterized by intraepidermal vesicles that result from severe ballooning of keratinocytes.

EPIDEMIOLOGY

Hand-foot-and-mouth disease is a common disease that chiefly affects children under 10 years of age. It usually occurs as an epidemic in day care centers and in schools between late spring and autumn.

CLINICAL FINDINGS

Cutaneous findings often are preceded by one or a few days of slight fever, malaise, diarrhea and a mouth that is so sore that the child may refuse to eat or drink. Painful vesicles, surrounded by zones of erythema, appear in the mouth, most frequently in the gingivolabial grooves, and on the tongue, buccal mucosa or hard palate. The blisters break quickly, leaving behind shallow, yellow–gray ulcerations. In about 20% of children affected, submandibular lymphadenopathy is palpable. Two-thirds of patients are affected by typical skin lesions on the fingers (Fig. 53.1), the toes, the sides of the feet (Fig. 53.2) or the palms and the soles. The vesicles are oblong or oval with gray roofs

and areolae of erythema. The vesicles tend to be aligned along lines formed by creases. The cutaneous lesions may vary in number from a few to over 50, and they may be asymptomatic or tender. Lesions generally resolve in 7–10 days.

HISTOPATHOLOGICAL FINDINGS

An intraepidermal vesicle marked by reticular alteration formed as a consequence of severe ballooning of keratinocytes, especially in the spinous zone (Fig. 53.3), is the histopathological hallmark of hand-foot-and-mouth disease.

AETIOLOGY AND PATHOGENESIS

Hand-foot-and-mouth disease is typically caused by enteroviruses, most commonly Coxsackievirus A16. The route through which the virus enters the body is the buccal mucosa or the intestinal tract. After infection of regional lymph nodes, the virus spreads to the mucosa and skin via the blood.

MANAGEMENT

Because the eruption and disease run a short course, only supportive care usually is necessary. In some children whose oral mucosae are severely affected, intravenous hydration may be required until intake of liquids by mouth is sufficient.

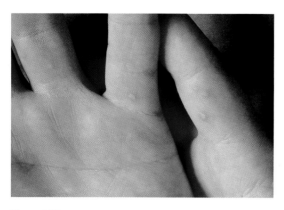

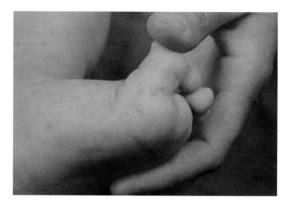

Figure 53.1
Hand-foot-and-mouth disease. There are numerous oblong vesicles surrounded by erythema on the palms. The vesicles have gray surfaces, a sign of necrosis of the epidermis.

Figure 53.2
Hand-foot-and-mouth disease. Oval, round and oblong papulovesicles are present on the medial aspect of the foot. A red rim surrounds some of the vesicles.

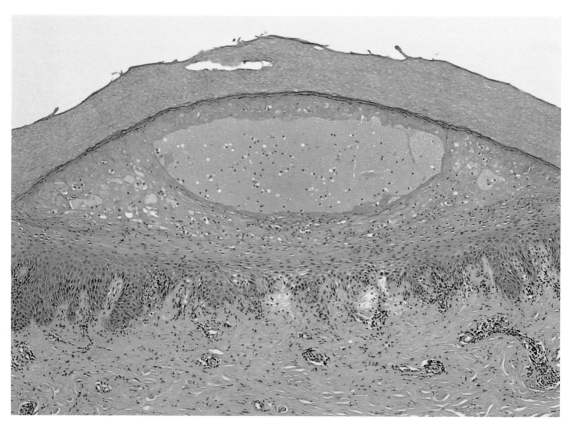

Figure 53.3
Hand-foot-and-mouth disease. There is intraepidermal vesicle within a zone of epidermal necrosis characterized by pink-staining keratinocytes that contrast with the blue-staining keratinocytes found in normal epidermis. Note the keratinocytes and pyknosis in the zone of necrosis.

54

HERPES SIMPLEX

The term herpes simplex refers to a group of infections caused by the human herpes simplex virus. The infections caused by herpes simplex virus type 1 and herpes simplex virus type 2 are conventionally classified as primary and recurrent. The cardinal clinical feature of herpes simplex is clusters of vesicles on top of red bases.

EPIDEMIOLOGY

Herpes simplex is one of the commonest infections of humans. Primary infection type 1 occurs mainly in infants and young children; primary infection type 2 occurs mainly after puberty. Primary infections are frequently asymptomatic or subclinical. Genital primary disease is more commonly symptomatic than oral.

CLINICAL FINDINGS

Primary infections caused by herpes simplex virus may manifest themselves clinically in six main ways:

- herpetic gingivostomatitis which is the most common primary infection caused by herpes simplex virus type 1 in children between the ages of 1 and 5 years. The infection causes high fever, sore throat and malaise. Painful vesicles in the oral cavity tend to become clustered and eventually form erosions on the buccal mucosa, tongue, palate and gingivae. Vesicles may appear on the lips and in the skin surrounding the lips. Profuse salivation,

fetid breath, dysphagia and regional lymphadenopathy are present in some patients. The oral manifestations usually resolve within 2–4 weeks;
- herpetic keratoconjunctivitis, which results from infections by herpes simplex virus type 1 and is usually expressed as severe conjunctivitis together with erythema, edema and vesiculation of the eyelids and periorbital skin (Fig. 54.1). Pain, photophobia and lacrimation are nearly constant symptoms. The cornea may be involved in about 10% of pediatric patients;
- herpes progenitalis, which refers to infection of genital region by herpes simplex virus type 2. Adolescents are most frequently affected. Local symptoms consist of pain and dysuria. Small vesicles, typically grouped, are present in early lesions. They become confluent, rupture and result in ulcers (Fig. 54.2);
- cutaneous inoculation, which is usually due to herpes simplex virus type 1 and most frequently involves the face, the hands and the feet (Fig. 54.3). A cluster of vesicles on an erythematous and edematous base is characteristic. Lesions may be marked by prominent local inflammation and by systemic symptoms, but these are usually less severe than mucous membrane manifestations. The term 'herpetic whitlow' refers to infection by herpes simplex virus of a hand or a finger;
- Kaposi's varicelliform eruption (eczema herpeticum), which appears in patients who suffer from cutaneous diseases such as atopic dermatitis or Darier's disease. About 5–10 days after the infective umbilicated vesicles appear, first in localized form at sites of already diseased skin and then in widespread array. The lesions usually

progress through vesicular, pustular, eroded and crusted stages (Fig. 54.4). Fever, malaise and generalized lymphadenopathy are present;

- neonatal herpes simplex, which results mostly from infection of an infant by herpes simplex virus type 2 during the passage through the birth canal during parturition. The most common skin lesions are vesicles on an erythematous base, which may eventuate in erosion or ulcerations. Skin manifestations may be localized to a particular site such as the head or buttocks or be disseminated.

Recurrent herpetic infections tend to occur as the same site as the primary one. The first indication of impending reactivation of infection is usually a sensation of burning or itching at the locus of the original infection. Vesicles appear and soon erode to heal without scars in 5–10 days. Recurrent infections are much less florid than the primary infection.

LABORATORY FINDINGS

Clinical diagnosis of primary infection by herpes simplex virus may be promptly confirmed by a Tzanck test on a vesicle. Primary herpes simplex viral infection is documented by obtaining serum and demonstrating seroconversion for herpes simplex virus antibodies by immunofluorescence techniques.

HISTOPATHOLOGICAL FINDINGS

Typical features of infection with herpes simplex virus may be found in epidermal and adnexal keratinocytes of lesions, namely, ballooned epithelial cells with steel-gray nuclei that show margination on their nucleoplasm (Figs 54.5 and 54.6). These changes are most marked within the spinous zone. The epithelial cells tend to become multinucleated, and intraepithelial blisters occur as a consequence of acantholysis.

ETIOLOGY AND PATHOGENESIS

Two major antigenic types of herpes simplex virus have been recognized:

- type 1, which is classically associated with facial infections;
- type 2, which mainly involves the genital area.

Primary infection occurs by direct exposure of a non-immune host to the virus, the route being mucocutaneous contact with an infected person. The virus then migrates and establishes a dormant infection within neuronal cells located in regional nerve ganglia. A hallmark of herpes simplex virus infection is its propensity for recurrence. Triggering factors may be events such as stress, exposure to sunlight, trauma or concurrent illness.

MANAGEMENT

Treatment should be started as soon as possible. Systemic acyclovir is the drug of choice and is effective in mucocutaneous infections, eczema herpeticum and neonatal herpes. Application of topical acyclovir is useful in the treatment of recurrent eruptions and in the prevention of corneal ulcers.

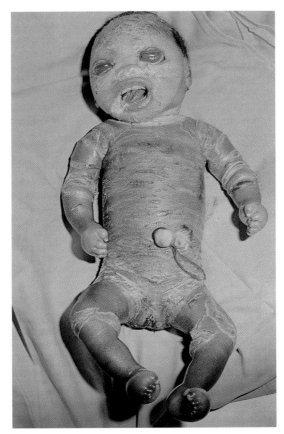

Figure 56.9
Congenital ichthyosis. Harlequin fetus. This fetus is characterized by deep fissures around armor-like plates that give the skin an appearance of an armadillo.

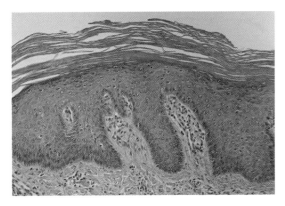

Figure 56.10
Congenital ichthyosis. Orthokeratosis in mostly compact array, a thick granular zone and epithelial hyperplasia are characteristic signs.

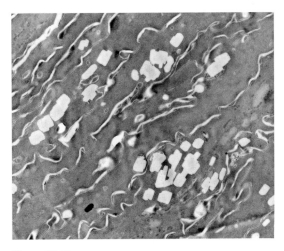

Figure 56.11
Congenital ichthyosis. Ultrastructure reveals groups of rod-shaped, electron-negative crystals in horny cells – pathognomonic markers of lamellar ichthyosis type II.

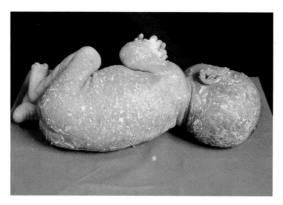

Figure 56.12
Netherton's syndrome. This newborn has widespread erythema covered by scales and scale-crusts. The diagnosis was made because the infant had bamboo hairs.

Figure 56.13
Netherton's syndrome. Double-edged desquamation at the periphery of the lesions is a distinctive finding.

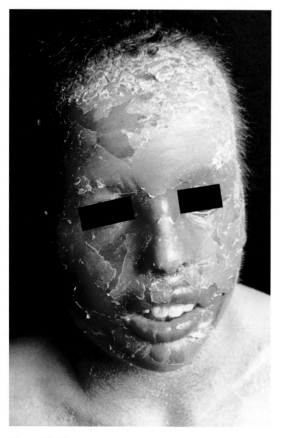

Figure 56.14
Netherton's syndrome. Diffuse erythema and large scales are prominent features. The hairs are short and sparse.

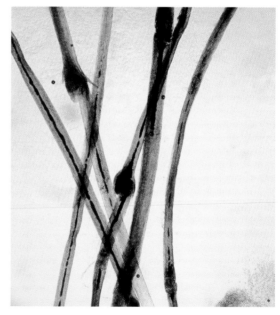

Figure 56.15
Netherton's syndrome. Bamboo joint swelling are typical of trichorrhexis invaginata.

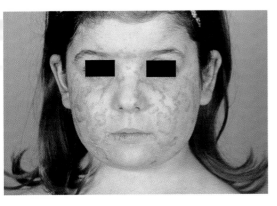

Figure 56.16
Erythrokeratodermia variabilis. Numerous lesions resemble those of gyrate erythema. Reddish papules form arcuate, annular and serpiginous shapes.

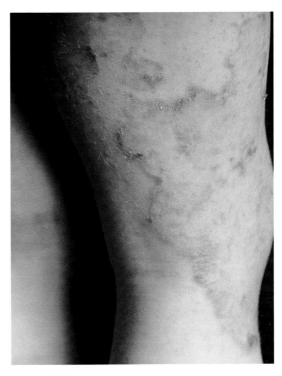

Figure 56.18 (*below*)
Erythrokeratodermia variabilis. A gently mamillated surface covered by orthokeratosis in basket-woven configuration is associated with hypergranulosis and epidermal hyperplasia, which are typical of this condition.

Figure 56.17
Erythrokeratodermia variabilis. The lesions are characterized by scalloped borders along which papules develop, some of which are scaly or crusted.

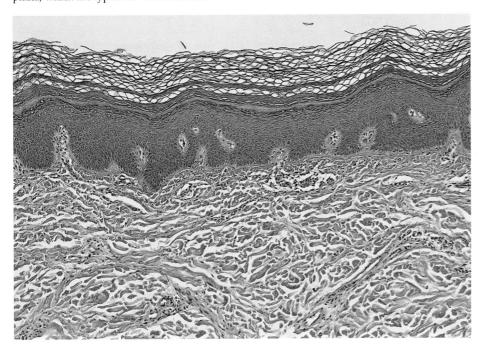

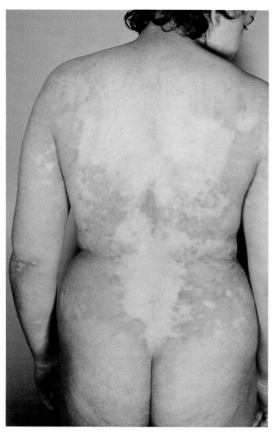

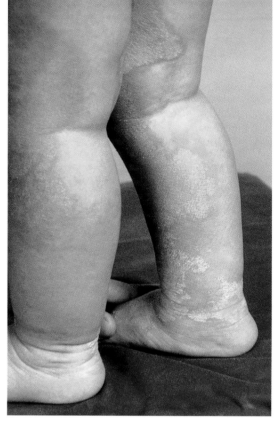

Figure 56.19
Symmetrical progressive erythrokeratodermia. The patient shows well-demarcated plaques with brownish bases and whitish scales. The lesions are distributed symmetrically.

Figure 56.20
Symmetrical progressive erythrokeratodermia. Brownish plaques that are surrounded by white scales characterize this condition.

INCONTINENTIA PIGMENTI

Incontinentia pigmenti is a complex, X-linked dominant disease characterized by four overlapping cutaneous stages and numerous neuroectodermal defects.

EPIDEMIOLOGY

Incontinentia pigmenti is rare but it occurs in all races and is usually present at birth. Approximately 95% of affected children are female, suggesting an X-linked mode of inheritance that is lethal in males.

CLINICAL FINDINGS

The first stage begins with erythema from which vesicles and, in time, bullae emerge (erythematous–bullous stage) (Fig. 57.1). Blisters may be present at birth, as may reddish macules and edematous papules. The blisters are at first filled with serum, which in time becomes turbid because of the incursion and disintegration of eosinophils. All of the lesions follow the whorled distribution of Blaschko's lines.

As the vesicular lesions slowly heal, they are replaced in the course of a few weeks by verrucous crusts and keratoses (verrucous stage) (Fig 57.2). The keratotic lesions thicken progressively and affect mainly the limbs, especially the fingers and the toes. Subungual keratoses may be painful.

As the verrucous lesions involute, whorled and linear zones of hyperpigmentation following Blaschko's lines appear (pigmentary stage). These zones occur mainly on the trunk, but the extremities are also often affected (Fig. 57.3). These hyperpigmented lesions represent post-inflammatory changes, even if parents aver that no inflammation occurred at these sites. The pigmented lesions usually fade gradually during late childhood or adolescence.

The fourth stage of incontinentia pigmenti consists of hypopigmented and atrophic skin lesions. These streaks are free of pilosebaceous units and sweat glands. The lack of results from long-term follow-up studies makes it difficult to establish whether hypopigmentation and atrophy represent a chronic evolution of the previous inflammatory or pigmentary stage or an independent feature of incontinentia pigmenti that can arise on previously clinically unaffected skin. Hypochromic and atrophic streaks and macules are distributed in a reticular pattern on the lower limbs or other region of the body, often visible at the legs in the unaware mothers and grandmothers of the child (Fig. 57.4). Although 80% of the vesicular and verrucous lesions come and go in a matter of weeks or months, the pigmented swirls my persist for decades. By puberty, however, they may clear. Hypochromic streaks can represent the only marker for incontinentia pigmenti in adulthood.

In about 80% of patients, associated abnormalities of the hair, the nails, the teeth, the eyes and the nervous system are present. Among these are cicatricial alopecia, nail dystrophy, cone-shaped teeth, anodontia, cataract, strabismus, seizures and mental retardation.

HISTOPATHOLOGICAL FINDINGS

The varied histopathological changes in incontinentia pigmenti parallel the variety of clinical findings. Histopathologically, the course of the disease process can be divided roughly into four stages – vesicular, pseudocarcinomatous, post-inflammatory and atrophic.

In the vesicular stage vesicles of incontinentia pigmenti are spongiotic and filled with eosinophils. Vesicles may be topped by mounds of scaly crusts that contain eosinophils. Beneath the vesicles is a sparse, superficial and deep, perivascular and interstitial infiltrate comprising mostly eosinophils (Fig 57.5).

The pseudocarcinomatous stage is typified by adnexal hyperplasia, especially infundibular, with numerous dyskeratotic cells. The lesion is covered by orthokeratosis and parakeratosis (Fig. 57.6).

Findings in the post-inflammatory stage, unlike those in the vesicular and pseudocarcinomatous stages, are not specific. Only a sprinkling of melanophages in a slightly thickened papillary dermis is noted (Fig. 57.7). Hypochromic lesions show epidermal atrophy and lack of adnexa, without significant melanocytic abnormalities. In the atrophic stage, the papillary dermis is thickened through fibroplasia, dermal papillae are effaced, and the epidermis is nearly devoid of rete ridges.

ETIOLOGY AND PATHOGENESIS

Incontinentia pigmenti is inherited in an X-linked, dominant pattern. The gene has been mapped on the long arm in region Xq 28, close to the factor VIII locus. The mutated gene is 'NEMO' (necrosis factor-kappa B essential modulator–IKKgamma). NEMO is required for the activation of the transcription factor necrosis factor-kappa B and is crucial in many inflammatory, immune and apoptotic pathways. The occurrence of the disease among men with normal karyotype XY may be caused by genetic mosaicism.

MANAGEMENT

No treatment has been helpful consistent in controlling the cutaneous lesions of incontinentia pigmenti. A thorough search of associated malformations is indicated in every affected child, because at least some of these malformations may be surgically correctable.

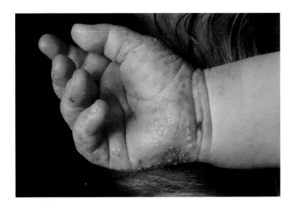

Figure 58.1
Infantile acropustulosis. Discrete pustules and yellow scaly crusts on acral skin are characteristic findings.

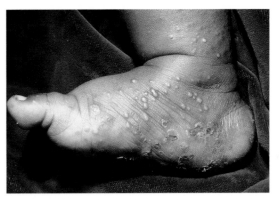

Figure 58.2
Infantile acropustulosis. These discrete pustules on the acra are diagnostic. Some of the pustules have resolved with erosions and ulcerations, and others have resolved with scaly crusts.

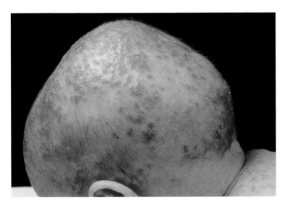

Figure 58.3
Infantile acropustulosis. Numerous rust-brown papules and papulopustules are present on the scalp.

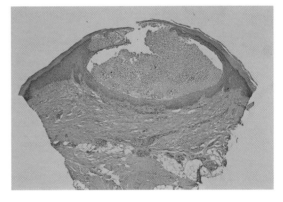

Figure 58.4
Infantile acropustulosis. The tense intraepidermal pustule is situated mostly in the spinous zone, but its roof is formed by the cornified layer.

INFANTILE DIGITAL FIBROMATOSIS

Infantile digital fibromatosis is a benign tumor of myofibroblasts that may be present at birth or appear after the first year of life. It involves the distal phalanx of a finger or a toe.

EPIDEMIOLOGY

Infantile digital fibromatosis is a rare disease.

CLINICAL FINDINGS

Infantile digital fibromatosis, also called 'recurring digital fibroma', is a dome-shaped neoplasm that arises on the distal phalanx of a finger or a toe (Figs. 59.1 and 59.2). Typically, the thumbs and great toes are spared. Lesions may reach a centimeter or more in diameter and, when large, become lobulated or pedunculated. Palpation reveals the lesions to be firm and seemingly adherent to underlying tissues. They range in color from that of skin through pink to red. Their surface is smooth. Spontaneous regression usually occurs in 2–3 years. Recurrences may be expected after surgical excision in 70% of the cases.

HISTOPATHOLOGICAL FINDINGS

Infantile digital fibromatosis is a dome-shaped lesion composed of interweaving fascicles of fibrous tissue that is marked by numerous, plump, oval fibrocytes and coarse, wiry bundles of collagen throughout the dermis and the subcutaneous fat (Figs 59.3 and 59.4). Eosinophilic globules are present within the cytoplasm of fibrocytes.

ETIOLOGY AND PATHOGENESIS

The cause of infantile digital fibromatosis is not known.

MANAGEMENT

Since the lesions of infantile digital fibromatosis tend to involute with time, treatment is not mandatory. When treatment is necessary, complete excision is the treatment of choice.

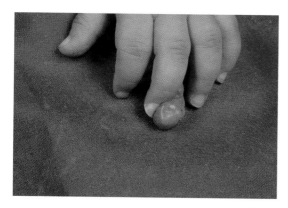

Figure 59.1

Infantile digital fibromatosis. This multilobulated, smooth, shiny, red–brown nodule is confined to a single digit.

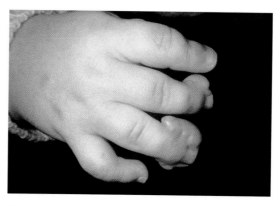

Figure 59.2

Infantile digital fibromatosis. Pink–blue , multilobulated nodules are present on the acral parts of two fingers in this infant.

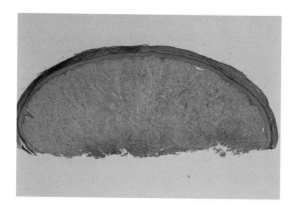

Figure 59.3

Figures 59.3. and 59.4

Infantile digital fibromatosis. This dome-shaped papule is characterized by an increased number of oval or spindle-shaped fibrocytes arranged in fascicles. Collagen, arrayed in thin bundles, is increased markedly.

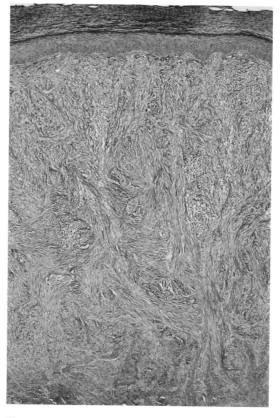

Figure 59.4

60 INFLAMMATORY LINEAR VERRUCOUS EPIDERMAL NEVUS

Inflammatory linear verrucous epidermal nevus (ILVEN) is a unilateral nevus that shows both inflammatory and psoriasiform features.

EPIDEMIOLOGY

The disease is rare. Females are four times as commonly affected as males. The age of onset is early, from birth to 4 years of age, with half of the patients developing the lesions in the first 6 months of life.

CLINICAL FINDINGS

ILVEN consists of discrete, erythematous, scaly, slightly verrucous papules that tend to coalesce and form linear plaques. The lesions are intensely pruritic (Figs 60.1 and 60.2). The lesions are unilateral; most commonly they occur on the left side of the body, especially on the left lower leg. They can be of any length and may involve the nails. Atrophy of the nails may occur. The course of this condition is chronic despite therapy.

HISTOPATHOLOGICAL FINDINGS

The histological appearance is inflammatory and psoriasiform (Fig. 60.3), with the following features:

- moderate acanthosis and papillomatosis;
- thickening of the epidermis;
- elongation of the rete ridges and dermal papillae;
- multiple small areas of spongiosis;
- exocytosis of neutrophils;
- alternating areas of parakeratosis and granulosis;
- perivascular lymphocytic infiltrate in the upper dermis.

ETIOLOGY AND PATHOGENESIS

The most plausible explanation for the existence of ILVEN is mosaicism.

MANAGEMENT

The treatment is unsatisfactory. The wide range of therapeutic trials include topical and intralesional corticosteroids, trichloracetic acid, cryotherapy, laser vaporization and surgical excision.

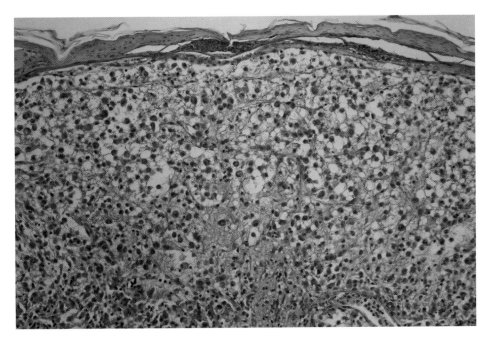

Figure 65.5

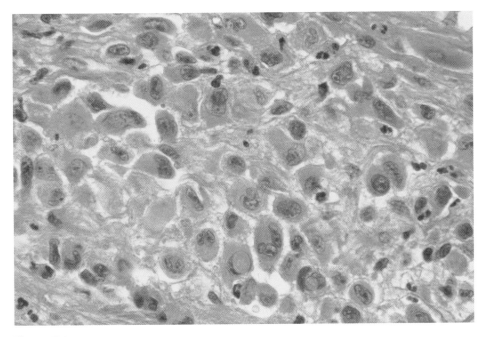

Figure 65.6

Figures 65.5 and 65.6
Langerhans cell histiocytosis. The papule shown here is characterized by an eroded, thinned epidermis covered by crust, beneath which is a dense, diffuse infiltrate of distinctive cells throughout the papillary dermis. These cells (Fig. 65.6) are characterized by bean-shaped nuclei and abundant eosinophilic cytoplasm.

66

LARVA MIGRANS

Larva migrans (or creeping eruption) is a broad term that describes the serpiginous, self-healing eruption caused by the accidental penetration of the skin by infective larvae of hookworms from various animals.

EPIDEMIOLOGY

Larva migrans is found most often in tropical and subtropical areas, especially coastal regions.

CLINICAL FINDINGS

Immediately after larvae penetrate the skin, the patient may experience a mild tingling sensation at the site of entry. The larvae can then lie quiet for weeks or months, or they may immediately begin to creep, with the production of single or multiple, pruritic, erythematous, raised tracks (Figs 66.1 and 66.2). The tracks are formed by papules and vesicles that contain serous fluid. These tunnel-like lesions may give rise to erosions. The leading portion of the track contains the larva, which advances at a rate of a few millimeters each day. The common entry sites are the feet, the hands, the buttocks, the calves, the arms and the thighs. The disease is self-healing in a few months, because humans are a 'dead-end' host.

LABORATORY FINDINGS

Eosinophilia has been observed.

HISTOLOGICAL FINDINGS

The histopathological findings are virtually indistinguishable from those caused by insect bites. There is a superficial and deep, perivascular and interstitial, mixed cell infiltrate made-up mostly of lymphocytes and eosinophils (Fig. 66.3). The papillary dermis is often edematous and the epidermis may house intercellular edema (spongiosis) and intracellular edema (ballooning).

ETIOLOGY AND PATHOGENESIS

The commonest causative agent is *Ancylostoma braziliensis*. Transmission is commoner in hot and rainy seasons because these conditions are appropriate for the development of the egg to the filiform larva stage. Warm sandy beaches contaminated with feces of dogs and cats represent a favorable condition for infection. The soil larvae may penetrate the skin through rhagades and hair follicles.

MANAGEMENT

Larva migrans usually does not require treatment because the worm dies spontaneously. However, this process may take several weeks to months, during which time the patient must endure both intensive pruritus and the discomforting sensation of a worm crawling through the skin. In children only topical treatment such as local freezing with liquid nitrogen, ethylchloride or dry ice under local anesthesia is recommended.

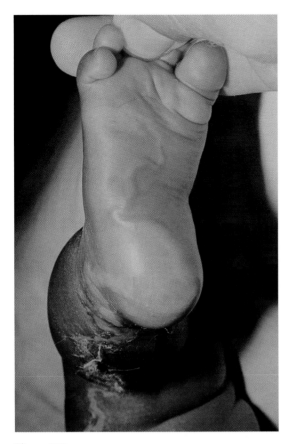

Figure 66.1
Larva migrans. This serpiginous track winds its way along the entire leg of this child.

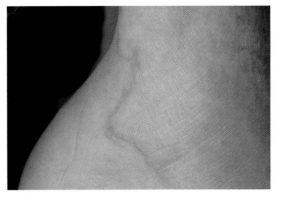

Figure 66.2
Larva migrans. An irregularly shaped, somewhat arcuate track formed by papules and vesicles is visible on the side of the foot.

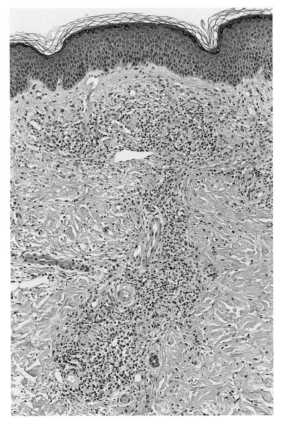

Figure 66.3
Larva migrans. Superficial and deep perivascular and interstitial mixed cell infiltrate of lymphocytes as well as eosinophils scattered among collagen bundles are a non-specific histopathologic finding.

67

LEISHMANIASIS

Cutaneous leishmaniasis (also known as oriental sore or Old World cutaneous leishmaniasis) is a granulomatous disease of the skin caused by *Leishmania tropica* complex (*Leishmania tropica* and *Leishmania major*) and *Leishmania aethiopica*, which are endemic in warm climates.

CLINICAL FINDINGS

The three clinical expressions of cutaneous leishmaniasis are acute, chronic and recidivans. Acute cutaneous leishmaniasis is more common in children. It begins as a single, asymptomatic, pink or red papule, 3–5 mm in diameter, at the site of a sandfly bite. Within 4–12 weeks, the papule evolves to a firm, inflamed, smooth, painful nodule (Fig. 67.1). The nodule enlarges progressively and eventually ulcerates and becomes crusted (Fig. 67.2). After removal, the crusts are soon replaced. After 5–12 months, the noduloulcerative lesions begin to regress from the center and, in time, resolve completely, leaving atrophic, irregular, disfiguring scars. Multiple lesions occasionally occur as the result of several bites by the sandfly that carries the protozoa. Superinfections occur in about 10% of patients, but their course is shorter and the lesions are smaller. The disease appears on the exposed areas of the body, especially the face and the arms.

The chronic form of leishmaniasis occurs only in elderly people, does not ulcerate and lasts for several years.

The recidivans form is rare and consists of new lesions that develop around scars at previously healed sites.

HISTOPATHOLOGICAL FINDINGS

Papules and nodules of acute leishmaniasis are characterized by dense, nodular and diffuse infiltrates composed mostly of histiocytes, neutrophils, and plasma cells. In the cytoplasm of the histiocytes reside numerous organisms of *Leishmania tropica* that appear as tiny blue dots in sections stained by hematoxylin and eosin (Figs 67.3 and 67.4). Such lesions may be eroded or ulcerated and covered by crusts.

ETIOLOGY AND PATHOGENESIS

Leishmania are protozoa of the family Trypanosomatidae. The parasite life cycle includes two forms, an extracellular, flagellated form (promastigote) in the vector and an intracellular non-flagellated form (amastigote) in infected mammals. Cutaneous leishmaniasis is caused by *L. tropica*, *L. major*, and *L. aethiopica*. These organisms are found only in cutaneous locations and do not tend to involve viscera. The most common vectors of the disease are *Phlebotomus papatasii* and *Phlebotomus sergenti*. The transmission occurs by the bite of an infected female sandfly that acquired its infection during a human blood meal 4–7 days previously. The commonest zoonotic reservoirs are gerbils and dogs. The incubation period varies from a few weeks to several months.

MANAGEMENT

The treatment of choice in children seems to be intralesional injection of methylglucamine antimoniate after local anesthesia. The lesions resolve promptly.

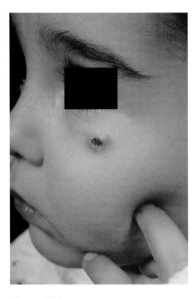

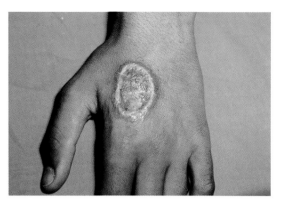

Figure 67.2
Acute cutaneous leishmaniasis. A large crater-like noduloulcerative lesion with a characteristic sloping edge.

Figure 67.1
Acute cutaneous leishmaniasis. A dark adherent crust is evident at the center of a firm nodule.

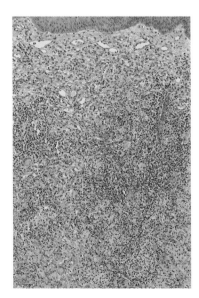

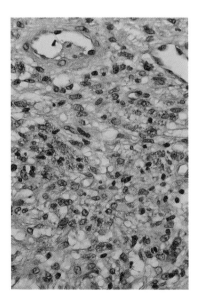

Figure 67.3

Figure 67.4

Figures 67.3 and 67.4
Acute cutaneous leishmaniasis. This patchy but diffuse infiltrate, made up mostly of mononuclear cells, harbors macrophages that contain organisms of Leishmaniasis. They are seen as tiny basophilic dots within the cytoplasm of the affected cells. Lymphocytes and numerous plasma cells are present together with macrophages.

68

LEIOMYOMA

Leiomyomas are benign neoplasms that are uncommon in children. They are composed of smooth muscle fibers. Three main types have been recognized, reflecting their different origins or differentiations:

- follicular leiomyoma, which arises from the arrector muscles of hair follicles;
- dartoic leiomyoma, which derives from the dartos muscle or the mamillary muscle of the nipple;
- angioleiomyoma, which originates from the smooth muscles of the blood vessels.

CLINICAL FINDINGS

Follicular leiomyoma appears as firm, red or dark brown nodules that vary in size from a few millimeters to 20 mm. The nodules are mainly situated on the trunk, the extremities and the head (Fig. 68.1). The number of the lesions may vary from few to several hundred. Adjacent tumors may coalesce to form plaques (Fig. 68.2). Single lesions have been observed. The characteristic feature of these tumors is paroxysmal pain induced by trauma, mild pressure or exposure to cold. This is the most frequent variety in children.

Dartoic leiomyoma is a solitary, deeply situated, non-painful nodule. Angioleiomyoma is a solitary, subcutaneous, well-circumscribed, asymptomatic nodule found on the extremities. After an initial period of growth, leiomyomas tend to become stationary. Pain, once established, tends to become progressively more severe.

HISTOPATHOLOGICAL FINDINGS

Leiomyomas have a silhouette of a benign neoplasm made up of myocytes (i.e. cells with elongated nuclei with blunt ends and vacuolated cytoplasm) (Figs 68.3 and 68.4).

MANAGEMENT

The tumors are typically benign, but since they are sometimes painful and also because malignant degeneration has been reported, surgical excision is recommended. Unfortunately, the tumor usually recurs.

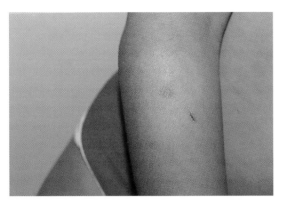

Figure 70.1
Indeterminate leprosy. Slightly hypopigmented macules with well defined borders.

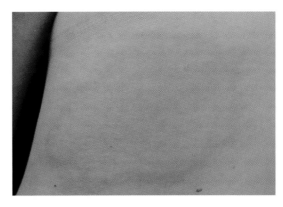

Figure 70.2
Tuberculoid leprosy. A large patch with central healing and a papular, erythematous edge.

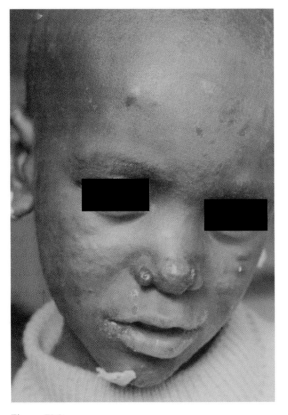

Figure 70.3
Lepromatous leprosy. The nodular eruption is widespread, but the face is the site of predilection. Few lesions on the limbs are ulcerated.

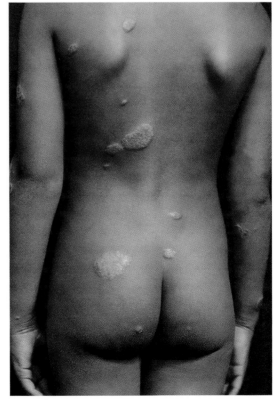

Figure 70.4
Borderline leprosy. Numerous plaques with clear-cut and elevated borders are distributed asymmetrically. The center of the plaques does not tend to heal.

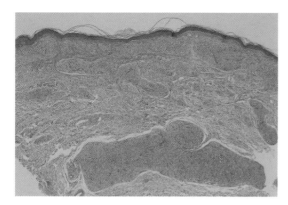

Figure 70.5

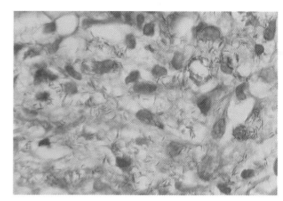

Figure 70.6

Figures 70.5 and 70.6
Lepromatous leprosy. The diagnosis of lepromatous leprosy is suggested by the appearance of elongated, snub-nosed aggregations consisting of pale histiocytes aligned along established vascular plexus. At higher magnification (Fig. 70.6), Ziehl–Nielsen stain reveals numerous acid-fast organisms within histiocytes.

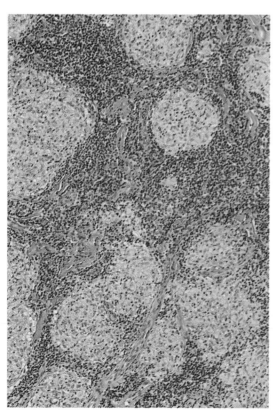

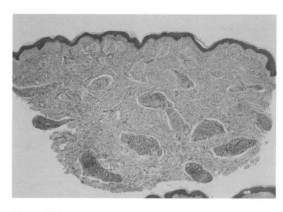

Figure 70.8
Borderline leprosy. This is borderline leprosy because the granulomas consists of both foamy and epithelioid histiocytes with a moderately dense infiltrate of lymphocytes around some of them.

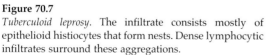

Figure 70.7
Tuberculoid leprosy. The infiltrate consists mostly of epithelioid histiocytes that form nests. Dense lymphocytic infiltrates surround these aggregations.

LICHEN AUREUS

Lichen aureus is a rare asymptomatic dermatosis of unknown origin, now classified into the group of pigmented purpuric dermatoses. The eruption consists of roundish or irregular, erythematous, purpuric papules, coalescent in patches, and mostly distributed on the limbs.

CLINICAL FINDINGS

Lesions of lichen aureus begin as red–purple, flat-topped papules of 1–3 mm in diameter. They are sometimes surmounted by fine, adherent scales. With time, the papules join to form plaques, and their color changes to shades of green–yellow, rust, bronze and even dark brown (Fig. 71.1). Failure of lesions at all stages to blanch on diascopy is characteristic. Plaques of lichen aureus are generally solitary, oval, well-circumscribed and small, usually not exceeding 30–50 mm in diameter. Rarely, plaques up to 200 mm in diameter may be seen, as may linear or multiple lesions. Lichen aureus is typically unilateral. Sites of predilection include the lower part of the leg, the thighs, the trunk and the upper extremities, in that order. Pruritus may be noted in early lesions, although most papules are asymptomatic. The lesions tend to regress in months or years.

HISTOPATHOLOGICAL FINDINGS

An infiltrate composed mostly of lymphocytes is present around the vessels of the superficial plexus and in band-like array in a thickened papillary dermis. Usually, the dermoepidermal junction is not obscured by the infiltrate. In early lesions, erythrocytes are extravasated in the papillary dermis (Fig. 71.2). Later, extravasated erythrocytes are few, but siderophages may be numerous throughout the thickened papillary dermis.

ETIOLOGY AND PATHOGENESIS

The etiology of the dermatosis is unknown. The postulated pathogenesis of lichen aureus is a capillaritis triggered by an infective focus that may sensitize the capillaries.

MANAGEMENT

Lichen aureus is unresponsive to topical or systemic treatment, but the disease is not disturbing and there is a slow tendency to spontaneous healing.

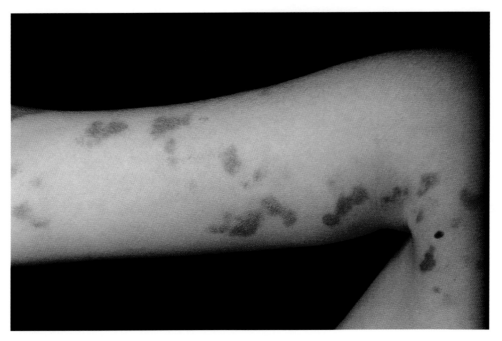

Figure 71.1
Lichen aureus. Asymptomatic, irregularly shaped rusty patches with a zosteriform pattern are seen here.

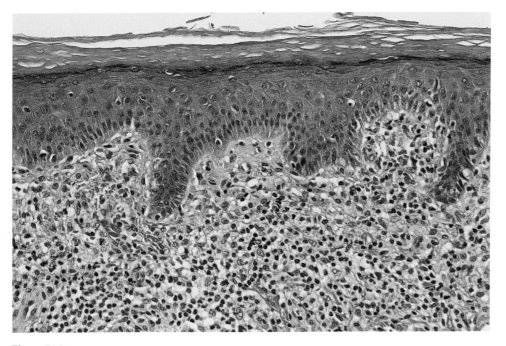

Figure 71.2
Lichen aureus. Lichen aureus is distinguished from other lichenoid dermatitides by the presence of numerous extravasal erythrocytes or siderophages (or both) within the lichenoid infiltrates of lymphocytes, as is evident in this section.

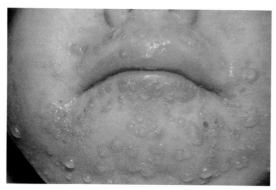

Figure 78.1
Linear immunoglobulin A dermatosis of childhood. The perioral region is a site of predilection. Many tense vesicles have ruptured and are weeping, resulting in serous crusts.

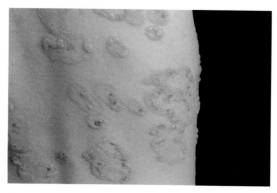

Figure 78.2
Linear immunoglobulin A dermatosis of childhood. Tense vesicles are present in arcuate and annular configurations that resemble rosettes. At the base of the vesicles, the skin is but slightly inflamed.

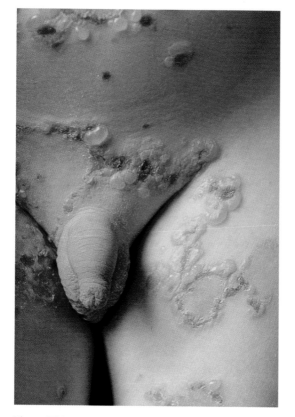

Figure 78.3
Linear immunoglobulin A dermatosis of childhood. Numerous tense vesicles are present, some in clusters, others in annular array. Residual hyperpigmentation is evident in the center of some of the rings. Note the hemorrhagic and yellowish crusts.

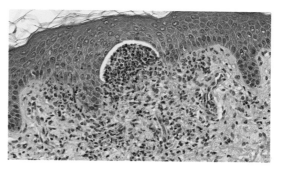

Figure 78.4
Linear immunoglobulin A dermatosis of childhood. The changes consist of a superficial perivascular and interstitial mixed cell infiltrate of neutrophils and eosinophils in focal collections at the tips of dermal papillae and in the subepidermal spaces.

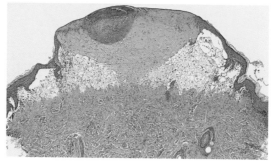

Figure 78.5
Linear immunoglobulin A dermatosis of childhood. The subepidermal blister has a necrotic epidermis as its roof and intact dermal papillae as its base. Within the blister itself and in the dermal papillae are collections of neutrophils.

LUPUS ERYTHEMATOSUS

Lupus erythematosus (LE) is a heterogeneous autoimmune disorder that includes a broad spectrum of clinical and laboratory findings. LE can be classified into four main forms: chronic LE with two varieties (discoid LE and lupus panniculitis), subacute cutaneous LE, systemic LE and neonatal LE.

DISCOID LUPUS ERYTHEMATOSUS

EPIDEMIOLOGY

Discoid LE is unusual in childhood. Its incidence in children ranges from 1 to 3%.

CLINICAL FINDINGS

The lesions may be located only on the face and external ear (localized discoid LE) or they may be diffuse (generalized discoid LE). They are characterized by well-defined erythematous, edematous, scaly patches with follicular plugging (Figs 79.1 and 79.2). The lesions have a tendency toward central clearing and, once healed, they usually leave atrophic, telangiectatic and pigmented scars. Lesions of the mucous membranes and scarring alopecia are extremely rare. The course is chronic, with remissions and relapses.

LABORATORY FINDINGS

The deposition of immunoglobulins and complement as a band or granular line along the dermoepidermal junction (lupus band

test) can be seen by direct immunofluorescence in more than 90% of specimens taken from affected areas, but not in clinically uninvolved skin.

HISTOPATHOLOGICAL FINDINGS

Discoid LE is characterized by typically thinned epidermis, vacuolar alteration of dermoepidermal junction, perivascular and periadnexal lymphocytic infiltrate and, often, deposits of mucin in the reticular dermis (Fig. 79.3).

MANAGEMENT

The treatment is similar to that for adults. Photoprotection by sunscreens together with topical or intralesional corticosteroids are recommended. Patients who do not respond to these measures may benefit from low doses of oral prednisolone (0.1–0.4 mg/day in the morning). Hydroxychloroquine has been used safely in pediatric patients at a dose of 7 mg/kg/day. An accurate ophthalmological examination is mandatory.

LUPUS ERYTHEMATOSUS PANNICULITIS (LUPUS PROFUNDUS)

EPIDEMIOLOGY

This form of discoid LE is typically a disease of middle age. No more than 20 cases have been reported in patients younger than 18 years.

CLINICAL FINDINGS

Lesions in the early stage of the disease consist of recurrent, deep, subcutaneous, small, non-tender nodules that arise primarily on the proximal portion of the limbs, the buttocks and the lower part of the back. The scalp, the face, and, more rarely, the legs may also be involved. Usually, the overlying skin is normal or slightly erythematous. Once healed, the lesions may leave cup-like depressions, attributable to subcutaneous atrophy, and considerable disfigurement (Fig. 79.4).

LABORATORY FINDINGS

Anti-nuclear antibodies can be detected in about 66% of pediatric cases and anti-nDNA antibodies in about 72%. Anti-cytoplasmic antibodies to Ro and La antigens are usually negative. The lupus band test of affected areas is positive in 70% of cases.

HISTOPATHOLOGICAL FINDINGS

LE panniculitis consists of patchy infiltrate of lymphocytes and plasma cells with lymphocytic nuclear 'dust' in concert with necrosis of adipocytes in fat lobules (Fig. 79.5).

MANAGEMENT

The treatment for patients with isolated LE panniculitis or with LE panniculitis associated with discoid lesions is similar to that for patients with chronic discoid DLE. Treatment with thalidomide was successful in a child in whom standard treatment failed.

SUBACUTE CUTANEOUS LUPUS ERYTHEMATOSUS

EPIDEMIOLOGY

Subacute cutaneous LE represents about 10% of all cases of LE with females affected more often than males.

CLINICAL FINDINGS

This LE subset may appear as erythematous, papular, scaly lesions (psoriasiform subacute cutaneous LE) or as annular erythematous, slightly scaling, polycyclic lesions. Atrophic scarring and follicular plugging are never observed; telangiectasia is often present. The disease is widespread, affecting the face, the shoulders, the upper trunk, the extensor part of the arm and the dorsum of the hand. Usually, photosensitivity is prominent. More than 50% of patients develop mild extracutaneous manifestations, such as fever, malaise and arthralgia. The systemic involvement is usually mild, so for the majority of patients the cutaneous manifestations represent the most important problem.

LABORATORY FINDINGS

Anti-dsDNA antibodies are present in low concentrations in the serum of about 30% of patients. Anti-Ro/SSA antibodies, a marker of neonatal LE, have been found in more than 65% of cases. Hypocomplementemia is rare. Lupus band test results are positive in only 50% of lesions and in 30% of uninvolved skin.

HISTOPATHOLOGICAL FINDINGS

The histological changes in subacute cutaneous LE are indistinguishable from those of early lesions of discoid LE, namely superficial, perivascular, lymphocytic infiltrates that partially obscure the dermoepidermal junction at the site of vacuolar alteration (Fig. 79.6). The epidermis is thinned, sometimes focally, but the cornified layer may be unaffected.

MANAGEMENT

Systemic therapy is required for most patients. The choice between antimalarial agents or moderate doses of oral prednisone in more severe cases, alone or in association, depends on the extent of the skin lesions, the severity of visceral involvement and the tolerance and responsiveness of the patient. Photoprotection and sun avoidance are also important to prevent worsening of skin lesions.

SYSTEMIC LUPUS ERYTHEMATOSUS

EPIDEMIOLOGY

The mean age of onset of systemic LE in children is 10 years. The disease is noted in people of all races and it is eight times more common in females than males.

CLINICAL FINDINGS

Cutaneous lesions of systemic LE can be classified as specific or non-specific. Specific lesions are characterized by an erythematous malar rash, commonly known as facial butterfly erythema, or by a scattered maculopapular edematous eruption (or both) (Figs 79.7 and 79.8). These lesions frequently arise after exposure to the sun and do not leave any skin atrophy. Telangiectasia of the palms, the fingers and mucous membranes may develop. Non-specific skin lesions are also important because they may be related to the degree of systemic LE activity. They consist of vasculitis, Raynaud's phenomenon (which affects about 33% of systemic LE patients), livedo reticularis, rheumatoid nodules, thrombophlebitis, diffuse non-scarring alopecia and calcinosis cutis. Vesicobullous eruptions are rare cutaneous manifestations of systemic LE (Fig. 79.9), but they may be the presenting and predominant skin lesions. Vesicles and bullae appear mostly on sites of sun exposure and the V portion of the chest, the upper part of the back, the hairline and the face. When skin lesions are present, evidence of multisystem involvement is prominent (arthritis, polyserositis, neurologic disorders and psychosis). Hematological and renal involvement are common. Fever,

malaise and weakness are frequent findings. The course of the disease is more aggressive in children than in adults.

LABORATORY FINDINGS

The erythrocyte sedimentation rate is consistently elevated. Polyclonal gammopathy, elevation of gammaglobulins and hypocomplementemia are frequent findings. Hemolytic anemia and leukopenia with lymphocytopenia or pancytopenia are common. Proteinuria, erythrocyturia and several types of urinary cellular casts may be present, their severity depending on the extent of renal disease. A high-titre anti-nuclear antibody test may be the most sensitive laboratory test for systemic LE, the nuclear fluorescence creating a homogeneous or peripheral pattern. Anti-dsDNA antibodies, often in high concentrations, are found in 60–80% of patients, whereas anti-Ro/SSA antibodies are found in only 25%. False-positive tests for syphilis and anti-cardiolipin antibodies also are noted. The lupus band test is positive in 95% of cases when using involved skin and in 75% of cases when using normal skin.

HISTOPATHOLOGICAL FINDINGS

The histological changes of systemic LE are indistinguishable from those of early lesions of subacute LE. In bullous systemic LE the blister is subepidermal and associated with neutrophils, neutrophilic nuclear dust and deposits of mucin in the reticular dermis (Fig. 79.10).

MANAGEMENT

The therapeutic schedule should be tailored to the severity of systemic involvement. For patients with less severe disease, anti-malarial and non-steroidal anti-inflammatory agents represent the first step in treatment. Prednisone (0.2–0.5 mg/day) given in a single morning dose or every other day to reduce toxicity, may be the second step. In the most severe cases, high doses of prednisone or oral immunosuppressive agents (or both) are used. Intravenous methylprednisolone pulses (15–30 mg/kg), intravenous cyclophosphamide, cyclosporine and plasmapheresis have been suggested as alternative therapeutic approaches in severe forms of systemic LE.

NEONATAL LUPUS ERYTHEMATOSUS

Neonatal lupus erythematosus is characterized by transient lupoid skin lesions or congenital heart block in an infant whose mother is affected by an autoimmune disorder or who bears anti-cytoplasmic antibodies and anti-Ro/SSA antibodies.

CLINICAL FINDINGS

Cutaneous lesions are present in approximately 85% of patients. They occur on exposed sites, such as the face (mainly the circumocular and temporal areas) and the scalp, often in response to ultraviolet light. Several kinds of lupoid lesions have been reported. The lesions are large, annular or circinate, sharply demarcated, erythematous macules, with no scaling or only light scaling (Figs 79.11 and 79.12). Healing leaves telangiectatic or dyschromic areas. Cardiac conduction defects (mainly congenital heart block) are present in about 54% of patients and begin *in utero*. Twenty-five per cent of patients with cardiac involvement have associated transposition of the great vessels and structural congenital heart defects. Other extracutaneous manifestations are autoimmune hemolytic anemia, thrombocytopenia, and hepatosplenomegaly. The eruption is self-limited, usually resolving within the first 6 months of life.

LABORATORY FINDINGS

Infants often fail to demonstrate serological abnormalities that are classically associated with systemic LE (including anti-nuclear antibodies and the LE cell test), despite the fact that they have anti-Ro/SSA antibodies and anti-La/SSB antibodies in their serum. These antibodies are also present in the mother. In affected infants, these antibodies disappear after about 12 months. The detection of these antibodies in the sera of newborns with lupoid cutaneous lesions or isolated congenital heart block is considered diagnostic of neonatal LE. The lupus band test is positive in only 50% of cases.

HISTOPATHOLOGICAL FINDINGS

The histopathological changes in neonatal LE are those of early discoid LE.

MANAGEMENT

No treatment is necessary in the absence of cardiac involvement. It is not known whether treatment of mothers during gestation is useful or harmful to fetuses with severe cardiac disease.

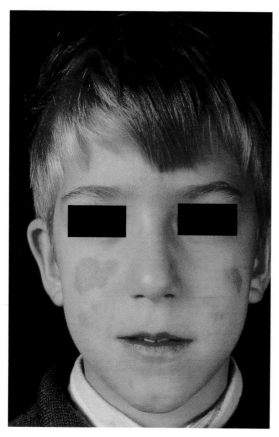

Figure 79.1
Discoid lupus erythematosus. Erythematous scaling plaques on the face of a 10-year-old boy.

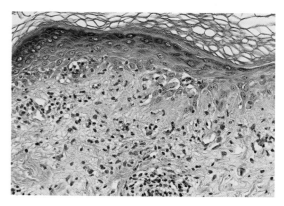

Figure 79.3
Discoid lupus erythematosus. This lesion can be inferred to be in its early stage because the infiltrate is superficial only, the cornified layers maintain its basket-woven configuration and the dermoepidermal junction is only slightly smudged by vacuolar alterations.

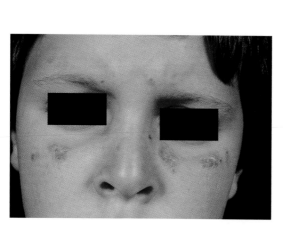

Figure 79.2
Discoid lupus erythematosus. Reddish papules covered by scaly crusts are present on the malar eminence and the forehead. Some of the crusts are hemorrhagic.

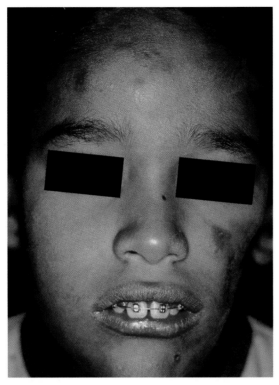

Figure 79.4
Lupus erythematosus panniculitis. Indurated plaques with central deeper atrophy are present on the left part of the face. The depression induced by the lesion is disfiguring. The erythematous scaling plaques on the forehead are characteristic of discoid LE.

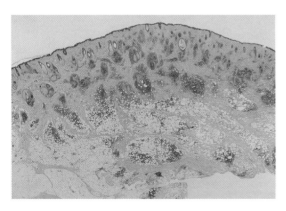

Figure 79.5
Lupus erythematosus panniculitis. The lesion involves both the dermis and the subcutaneous fat. In the latter location, patchy infiltrates of lymphocytes and plasma cells are associated with necrosis of adipocytes.

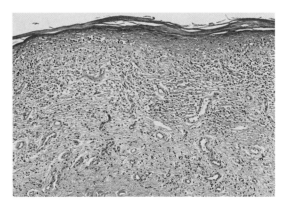

Figure 79.6
Subacute lupus erythematosus. Superficial and perivascular lymphocytic infiltrate partially obscure the dermoepidermal junction at the site of vascular alteration.

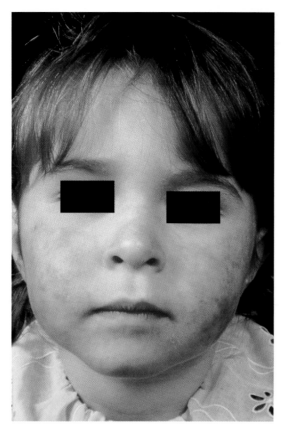

Figure 79.7
Systemic lupus erythematosus. The lesions consist of erythematous, slightly edematous, poorly demarcated patches. Scaling and atrophy are absent.

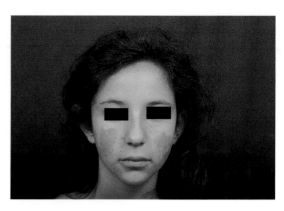

Figure 79.8
Systemic lupus erythematosus. Typical malar rash.

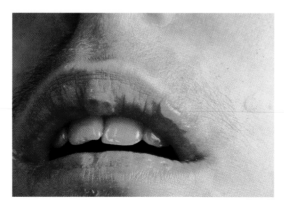

Figure 79.9
Systemic lupus erythematosus. Vesicles and small blisters appeared on the lips of this patient after sun exposure.

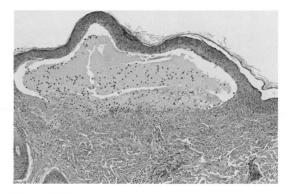

Figure 79.10
Bullous systemic lupus erythematosus. The subepidermal blister houses abundant plasma cells and many neutrophils. Neutrophils and neutrophilic nuclear 'dust' are also present in dermal papillae and at the base of the blister.

MALIGNANT MELANOMA

Malignant melanoma is a malignant neoplasm that originates from melanocytes. Malignant melanoma usually begins as a proliferation of atypical melanocytes in the epidermis that extends into the dermis and subcutaneous tissue, sites from which it may metastasize.

EPIDEMIOLOGY

About 0.4% of malignant melanomas occur in prepubertal children. They may appear at any age and may be present at birth.

CLINICAL FINDINGS

Malignant melanomas in infants and children arise mainly in association with pre-existing congenital types of melanocytic nevi, especially the large, hairy kind (Fig. 83.1). Only rarely do these lesions arise *de novo* (i.e. in the absence of a melanocytic nevus). Malignant melanoma may evolve from macules to patches (Fig. 83.2) or from macules to papules to nodules and tumors. Whatever the anatomical site, melanomas tend to be asymmetrical, scalloped or notched at the periphery, and variegate in color, especially in nuances of brown, ranging from tan to black. When this neoplasm undergoes regression, zones of white or off-white appear, followed by a patch or plaque. It is exceedingly difficult to recognize the development of malignant melanoma within a large, hairy congenital nevus because such lesions usually do not have the features of malignant melanomas that arise *de novo*. By the time it is detected, the lesion is usually an indistinct nodule or tumor in the substance of the nevus.

The course of malignant melanoma is as unpredictable in children as it is in adults. Some malignant melanomas grow rapidly and metastasize quickly, whereas others are more indolent and do not metastasize for many years. Thick malignant melanomas with large volumes of neoplastic cells tend to metastasize more readily.

HISTOPATHOLOGICAL FINDINGS

The diagnostic findings of malignant melanoma, whatever the anatomical site, are asymmetry, poor circumscription, failure of maturation of melanocytes with progressive descent into the dermis, nests of melanocytes within the epidermis that vary in size and shape, and nests in the epidermis that have become confluent at least in some foci (Figs 83.3 and 83.4). Cytologically, features of importance are nuclear atypia, an increased number of mitotic figures (especially near the base of the neoplasm) and the presence of necrotic neoplastic cells. Another diagnostic clue is the presence of atypical pagetoid melanocytes arranged in a pagetoid pattern within the epidermis (i.e. neoplastic cells with large atypical nuclei and abundant pale-staining cytoplasm that contain dusty melanin). Pagetoid melanocytes in a pagetoid pattern are virtually diagnostic of malignant melanoma.

ETIOLOGY AND PATHOGENESIS

Racial traits such as fair skin and a tendency to sunburn rather than to tan, together with intense sunlight exposure have been advocated as risk factors for malignant melanomas in adults. The importance of these factors on the development of malignant melanoma in children has not been determined. Many malignant melanomas in children arise in large congenital melanocytic nevi, and according to various studies, the lifetime expected frequency of development of malignant melanoma in such nevi ranges from 4.6 to 14%. The mechanism whereby malignant melanomas develop in pre-existing melanocytic nevi has yet to be delineated. The familial occurrence of melanoma is well established. Children in these melanoma-prone families typically develop more acquired melanocytic nevi (Clark's nevi) than is common in children their age.

MANAGEMENT

Therapy for primary cutaneous melanoma is complete excision of the neoplasm. If excision occurs before the melanoma has metastasized, no matter how narrow the margin, the patient is cured. If, however, metastasis occurs before the definitive surgical procedure, the patient is likely to die of metastatic melanoma, no matter how wide and how deep the blade of the surgeon is carried. No evidence supports the contention that wider excisions for thicker lesions has merit. The usefulness of studying a regional lymph node (sentinel lymph node) is controversial.

Chemotherapy and various forms of immunotherapy have proven as ineffective in children as they are in adults. The inadequacy of available treatment for metastatic melanoma underlines the importance of early diagnosis and prompt surgical treatment of malignant melanomas in children.

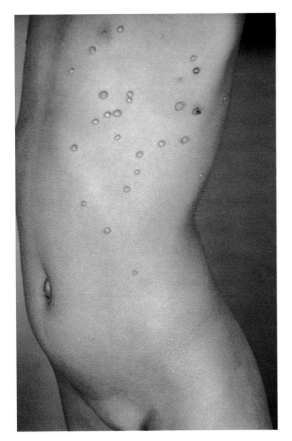

Figure 86.1

Molluscum contagiosum. These reddish-brown, discrete papules have a central dell that contains cornified cells.

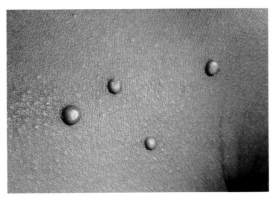

Figure 86.2

Molluscum contagiosum. These hemispheric brownish papules have a distinct central umbilication.

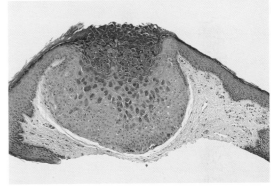

Figure 86.3

Molluscum contagiosum. This dome-shaped lesion consists of a hyperplastic infundibulum, the ostium of which is plugged by corneocytes. Within the majority of epithelial cells in this bulbous epithelium are molluscum bodies. These structures, which are confined to the cytoplasm, are ovoid and consist of amphophilic granular material. Note that molluscum bodies in the cornified layer stain more darkly than those in the viable epithelium.

MUCINOSIS

The cutaneous mucinoses consist of a hetero-geneous group of diseases characterized by accumulation of mucin in the dermis, either focally or diffusely.

EPIDEMIOLOGY

Primary cutaneous mucinoses are extremely rare in the pediatric population.

CLINICAL FINDINGS

Cutaneous mucinosis of infancy

Cutaneous mucinosis of infancy is character-ized by the eruption of multiple, small (1–2 mm), pale, opalescent, firm papules. These lesions, which are densely grouped, are distributed symmetrically on the elbows. Solitary lesions may be seen on the arms and the dorsum of the hands.

Self-healing juvenile cutaneous mucinosis

Self-healing juvenile cutaneous mucinosis (Fig. 87.1) consists of the rapid onset on the face, the trunk and the limbs of asymptomatic papules that merge into infiltrated, non-tender plaques. Deep nodules may be observed on the face and periarticular regions. Signs of arthritis are present in the knees, the elbows and the fingers. Regression occurs in a few months.

Follicular mucinosis

Follicular mucinosis appears as follicular papules mimicking chronic folliculitis. Frequently, papules merge into erythematous plaques (Fig. 87.2) that may or may not be alopecic, and their surface may show empty follicular openings. Sites of predilection are the face and the neck. The lesions may persist for years.

Acral persistent papular mucinosis

Acral persistent papular mucinosis is identi-fied by the asymptomatic eruption of multi-ple, white, translucent persistent papules of 2–5 mm in diameter that are located symmet-rically on the back of the hands (Fig. 87.3), the forearms and the wrists.

HISTOPATHOLOGICAL FINDINGS

Cutaneous mucinosis of infancy, self-healing juvenile cutaneous mucinosis and acral persistent papular mucinosis are character-ized by deposits of mucin in the papillary or upper reticular dermis, which leads to separa-tion and fragmentation of collagen bundles.

The main histological changes in follicular mucinosis are deposits of mucin that are located mainly in the outer root sheet together with a mixed inflammatory cell infiltrate around and within the follicular epithelium (Fig. 87.4).

ETIOLOGY AND PATHOGENESIS

The initial stimulus that induces an increase and accumulation of acid glycosaminoglycans (mucin) and fibroblast proliferation remains unknown in primary cutaneous mucinoses. In these diseases, mucin appears to consist of hyaluronic acid and dermatan sulfate.

MANAGEMENT

No treatment is effective.

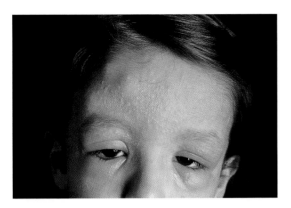

Figure 87.1
Cutaneous self-healing mucinosis. The upper part of the face is covered by tiny, skin-colored papules, some in linear array. Two deep nodules are evident on the forehead, and the eyelids are swollen.

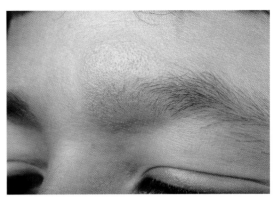

Figure 87.2
Follicular mucinosis. A nummular erythematous plaque involves the forehead and the eyebrows, inducing partial alopecia.

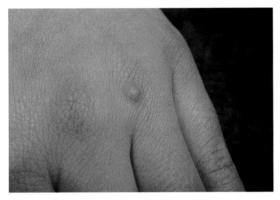

Figure 87.3
Acral persistent papular mucinosis. A white, translucent, persistent papule on the back of the hand of a 13-year-old girl.

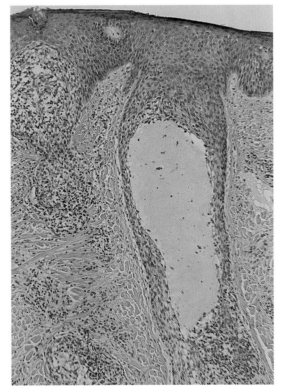

Figure 87.4
Follicular mucinosis. Abundant deposits of mucin are observed in the outer root sheet of most of the follicles in this section. A moderately dense, mixed inflammatory cell infiltrate composed mostly of lymphocytes and histiocytes is present around and within the follicular epithelium.

NECROBIOSIS LIPOIDICA

Necrobiosis lipoidica is a degenerative disease of the connective tissue characterized by asymptomatic, slightly depressed, atrophic plaques that are usually located over the anterior surface of the legs.

EPIDEMIOLOGY

Necrobiosis lipoidica is uncommon in the pediatric age group and is closely associated with diabetes mellitus. The disease is three times commoner in women than men.

CLINICAL FINDINGS

Skin lesions of necrobiosis lipoidica demonstrate a distinctive evolution. The process begins with 1–3 mm, red–brown, firm papules that coalesce and expand slowly to form large, oval or irregular plaques. The border of the plaques is often violaceous, slightly elevated and sharply demarcated; the center is depressed or atrophic with a waxy, yellow, translucent surface (Figs 88.1 and 88.2). Multiple telangiectases are easily seen through the atrophic epidermis. Variable amounts of scaling may be present. These plaques are alopecic, hypohidrotic and sometimes partially or completely anesthetic. In 85–90% of patients, lesions arise on the pretibial area and are often bilateral. In the remaining patients, necrobiosis lipoidica may occur on the scalp, the face, the arms or the trunk. The commonest complication is recurrence of ulceration after trauma. The disease has a chronic course with periods of waxing and waning of the lesions. Spontaneous resolution has been reported in about 15% of cases.

HISTOPATHOLOGICAL FINDINGS

Fully developed lesions are characterized by the involvement of the entire reticular dermis with a lymphoplasmocytic perivascular infiltrate, histiocytes arrayed in palisades and extensive degeneration of collagen in the center of the granuloma (Figs 88.3 and 88.4). In advanced lesions, sclerosis replaces the collagen degeneration and the number of inflammatory cells decreases.

ETIOLOGY AND PATHOGENESIS

The etiopathogenesis of necrobiosis lipoidica is still unknown. Many experts believe that the primary event is diabetic microangiopathy, resulting in collagen degeneration attributable to vascular occlusion. The demonstration of immunoglobulin M, immunoglobulin A and complement (C3) deposition in vessel walls raises the possibility that the primary event is an antibody-mediated vasculitis. Trauma is considered a triggering factor rather than a causative factor.

MANAGEMENT

Treatment of necrobiosis lipoidica is usually not satisfactory. It is useful to protect the legs with occlusive bandaging to avoid trauma. Corticosteroid injections into active areas may clear some lesions, but atrophy may occur.

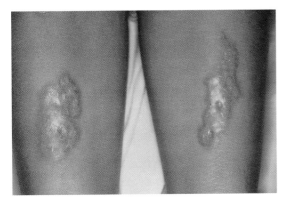

Figure 88.1
Necrobiosis lipoidica. Bilateral, irregular, yellow–red atrophic plaques with a waxy translucent surface, coursed by telangiectatic vessels and with violaceous borders are present on the anterior surface of the legs.

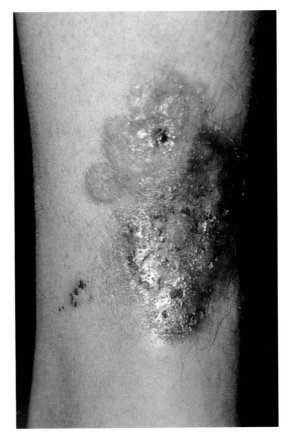

Figure 88.2
Necrobiosis lipoidica. These plaques have different sizes and shapes and tend to confluence. Some borders are scalloped and sharply circumscribed. The plaques situated superiorly have a yellowish cast as well as zones that are pink and purple. The plaque found inferiorly is dark purple and ulcerated.

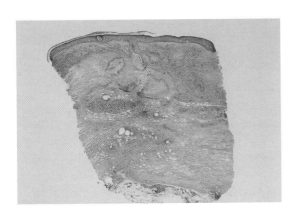

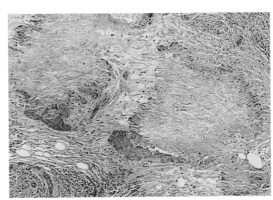

Figure 88.3

Figure 88.4

Figures 88.3 and 88.4
Necrobiosis lipoidica. At scanning magnification the patchy pink zones represent degeneration of collagen. At the periphery of these zones, histiocytes are arrayed in a palisade (Fig. 88.4). A lymphoplasmocytic infiltrate is present around blood vessels in the dermis and the subcutaneous fat.

NEUROFIBROMATOSIS

Neurofibromatosis is an autosomal-dominant disease. It is characterized by changes in the skin, the nervous system, the bones and the endocrine glands. Four forms are now recognized: peripheral neurofibromatosis (von Recklinghausen's disease or NF1), acoustic neurofibromatosis (NF2), segmentary neurofibromatosis, and multiple café-au-lait spots without associated findings.

Epidemiology

Neurofibromatosis is one of the commonest genodermatoses, with an estimated incidence of 1 in 3000 live births. Males are slightly more often affected than females.

Clinical findings

Von Recklinghausen's disease is characterized by three hallmark features – multiple café-au-lait spots, multiple neurofibromas, and Lisch nodules. Café-au-lait macules are present in 99% of patients. They are usually present at birth or become apparent during the first months of life and frequently represent the first sign of the disease. The spots are regularly circumscribed, light or dark brown patches. They vary in diameter from 2 mm to more than 150 mm, and are randomly distributed over the body surface. The presence of at least six café-au-lait macules that exceed 5 mm before puberty or 15 mm after puberty in broadest diameter are considered pathognomonic for neurofibromatosis. Freckling, with clusters of hyperpigmented macules about 2 mm in diameter in intertrigi-

nous areas such as the axillary vault (Crowe's sign), is an important sign (Fig. 89.1).

Neurofibromas occur in childhood independent of café-au-lait spots; they are usually widespread except for the palmoplantar surfaces. They may be superficial or subcutaneous. The superficial tumors are soft, pink, sessile or pedunculated lesions that vary in size and number. The subcutaneous tumors may occur as violaceous nodules along a peripheral nerve or as deeper, large plexiform masses (Fig. 89.2).

Pigmented hamartomas of the iris (Lisch nodules) are present in 90% of patients over 12 years of age and in more than 30% of patients of 6 years of age or older. They are asymptomatic but increase in number with age and are important for diagnosis, especially when other clinical manifestations are not prominent. Additional cutaneous signs include hypopigmented lesions and xanthogranulomas.

Neurological involvement is present in 40% of patients. Neural crest tumors include gliomas, meningiomas, astrocytomas, neuromas, pheochromocytomas, neurofibrosarcomas and malignant schwannomas. Optic chiasmatic glioma is a particularly frequent finding in children. Intellectual handicaps, speech impediments and seizure disorders depend on the degree of central nervous system involvement. Skeletal abnormalities such as macrocephaly, kyphoscoliosis, bone cysts and pseudoarthroses of long bones have been found in almost 50% of patients. Endocrinological dysfunctions of various types and vascular deformities may complete the clinical picture. The course is variable, but usually it is slowly progressive.

Acoustic neurofibromatosis is characterized by bilateral acoustic neuromas, the frequent presence of other central nervous system tumors such as astrocytomas, the paucity of café-au-lait spots (which are seen in less than 50% of cases) and peripheral neurofibromas (which are seen in less than 20% of cases), and the absence of Lisch nodules and skeletal abnormalities.

Segmental neurofibromatosis is characterized by café-au-lait spots or cutaneous neurofibromas localized to a segment of the body with a unilateral dermatomal distribution.

Multiple café-au-lait spots is a subtype of neurofibromatosis. Affected patients have only multiple café-au-lait spots, which are more than 15 mm in broadest diameter, inherited as an autosomal-dominant trait. There are no associated Lisch nodules, neurofibromas, skeletal problems or any of the other characteristic features described above.

HISTOPATHOLOGICAL FINDINGS

Neurofibromas are sharply circumscribed, benign neoplasms that consist of delicate fibrillary bundles of collagen accompanied by cells with wavy nuclei (Figs 89.3 and 89.4). Café-au-lait spots consist of typical melanocytes in normal numbers situated at the dermoepidermal junction.

ETIOLOGY AND PATHOGENESIS

Von Recklinghausen's disease is an autosomal-dominant disease with no race predilection, a penetrance that approaches 100%, and extremely variable expression. About 50% of cases represent spontaneous mutations. The von Recklinghausen's disease gene has been localized to the proximal long arm of chromosome 17 (NF1 gene) and the gene of acoustic neurofibromatosis has been localized to the long arm of chromosome 22. Segmental neurofibromatosis probably results from a postzygotic somatic mutation, with minimal risk of familial transmission of the disease. The pathogenesis of lesions in all forms of neurofibromatosis is still unknown.

MANAGEMENT

The two most important aspects of treatment are genetic counselling and surgical excision of neurofibromas when necessary (because of rapid growth, pain or functional or esthetic problems) and possible.

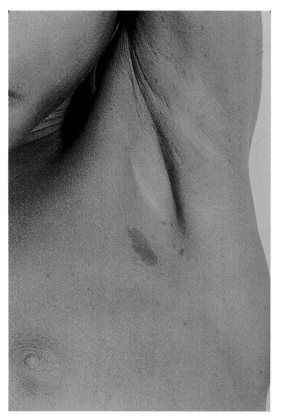

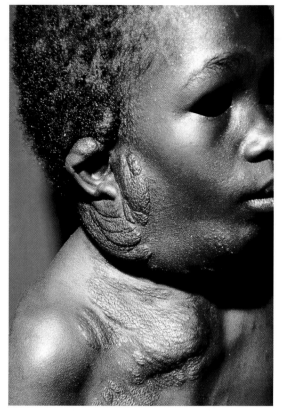

Figure 89.1
Neurofibromatosis. Crowe's sign: hyperpigmented macules and a café-au-lait spot in the axilla. These lesions are sometimes referred incorrectly as axillary freckles.

Figure 89.2
Neurofibromatosis. The cerebriform lesions around the ear are characterized histologically by the changes of a plexiform neurofibroma.

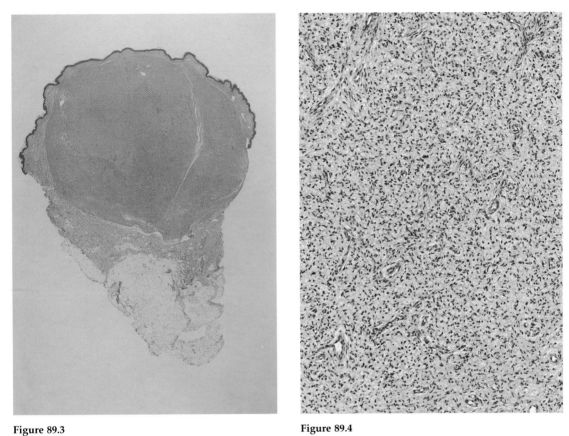

Figure 89.3 **Figure 89.4**

Figures 89.3 and 89.4

Neurofibroma. This neoplasm is benign; it is symmetrical and well circumscribed, and it has smooth borders. It is a neurofibroma because its numerous cells have oval and wavy nuclei, the collagen associated with it is fibrillary, and numerous venules course throughout it. Abundant mucin, seen as granular basophilic material, is present within the stroma (Fig. 89.4).

NEVUS ACHROMICUS

Nevus achromicus (also called nevus depigmentosus) is a rare, congenital, non-familial, stationary, hypomelanotic macular lesion. The lesion is often located on the trunk.

EPIDEMIOLOGY

The incidence of nevus achromicus is difficult to estimate because the clinical problems are often not sufficient to induce patients to contact a dermatologist. In the authors' opinion it is common.

CLINICAL FINDINGS

Nevus achromicus consists of hypopigmented areas that are irregular in shape and size, have geographical margins, and change from pale to white (Fig. 90.1). Lesions usually involve the trunk and the proximal extremities, but the face and the neck may also be affected. The nevus is often unilateral or circumscribed, or has a dermatomal pattern, but it may be systematized. Theoretically present at birth, it may become evident only after several months or even years of life.

The systematized variant of nevus achromicus corresponds to incontinentia pigmenti achromians or hypomelanosis of Ito. This disorder may be subdivided into a cutaneous form, in which the disease is limited to pigmentary changes and sweating abnormalities, and a neurocutaneous form, with severe nervous system defects and bony abnormalities in addition to hypopigmentation. In the systematized variant, lesions manifest themselves as a hypopigmented band and whorl on the trunk and extremities, with a bizarre pattern similar to that of incontinentia pigmenti (i.e. following Blaschko's lines). These lesions tend to progress initially and then remain stable.

HISTOPATHOLOGICAL FINDINGS

Normal melanocytes are present in the epidermis, which is normal except for decreased amounts of melanin within keratinocytes (Fig 90.2).

ETIOLOGY AND PATHOGENESIS

Nevus achromicus seems to be the consequence of decreased synthesis and abnormal transfer of melanosomes.

MANAGEMENT

No effective treatment is available.

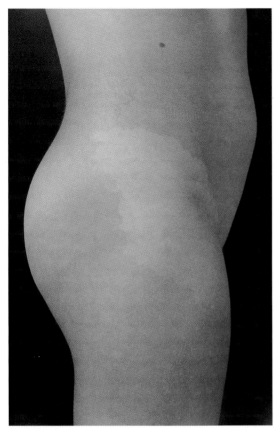

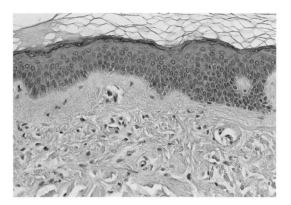

Figure 90.2
Nevus achromicus. This patch is clinically dramatic but histopathologically unremarkable. In fact, no abnormalities are detectable.

Figure 90.1
Nevus achromicus. This broad, irregularly shaped, hypopigmented patch is congenital and unilateral and has not enlarged.

91 NEVUS LIPOMATOSUS CUTANEOUS SUPERFICIALIS

Nevus lipomatosus cutaneous superficialis is an idiopathic hamartoma characterized by mature ectopic adipose tissue in the dermis.

EPIDEMIOLOGY

Nevus lipomatosus cutaneous superficialis is very rare.

CLINICAL FINDINGS

Two clinical variants have been described, a solitary form and a multiple form. The multiple form (the classic form originally described by Hoffman and Zurhelle) consists of aggregates of soft, asymptomatic, skin-colored or yellow, elevated papules or nodules that sometimes coalesce into plaques with cerebriform surfaces (Fig. 91.1). Such plaques vary in size up to 80 mm by 150 mm. The predominant sites for lesions is the pelvic girdle, particularly the gluteal, sacral, and coccygeal regions, and the upper part of the posterior aspects of the thighs. In a few cases, lesions are confined to the abdominal, thoracic, and lumbar regions, the extremities and the scalp. Only rarely do the nodules extend across the midline. Solitary lesions may be dome-shaped, sessile or pedunculated, and solitary lesion have been reported at sites other than those of the classic form, including the knee, the axilla, the arm and the scalp. Onset is at birth, during childhood or in adolescence. Once formed, the lesions remain unchanged or enlarge for many years.

HISTOPATHOLOGICAL FINDINGS

Nevus lipomatosus cutaneous superficialis is characterized by sheets of adipocytes through the dermis and caricatures of them in the subcutaneous fat, which is intersected by thickened, haphazardly arranged septa. These septa consist of thickened bundles of collagen, which are sometimes associated with deposit of mucin (Fig. 91.2)

ETIOLOGY AND PATHOGENESIS

The cause of nevus lipomatosus cutaneous superficialis is unknown.

MANAGEMENT

Treatment, if required, is by surgical excision.

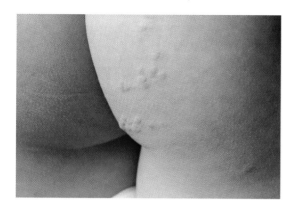

Figure 91.1
Nevus lipomatosus cutaneous superficialis. Some of the numerous skin-colored papules are arranged in clusters. The buttocks is a site of predilection.

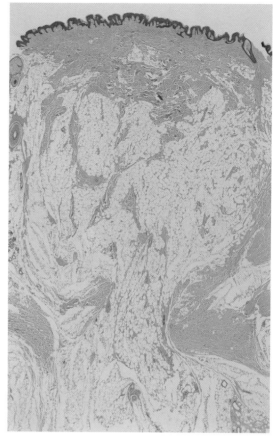

Figure 91.2
Nevus lipomatosus cutaneous superficialis. Much of the lower half of the dermis has been replaced by collections of adipocytes that vary in size and shape. The subcutaneous fat is also altered by an increased number of haphazardly arranged septa. Lobules of adipocytes are not intersected by thin fibrous septa in the manner of normal subcutaneous fat; instead, the connective tissue elements, both fibrous and adipose, are organized in a way that has completely changed the architecture of the subcutaneous fat. The collagen bundles that form aberrant septa are thicker than those within normal fibrous septa, and many of the lobules of adipocytes are accompanied by abundant mucin, seen as granular, probably basophilic material.

NEVUS SEBACEUS

Nevus sebaceus is a localized hamartoma of the epidermis and the pilosebaceous units and, occasionally, of the ectopic apocrine glands.

EPIDEMIOLOGY

The lesion is present in 0.3% of all neonates, with an equal incidence in males and females. In most cases nevus sebaceus is seen at birth but it may be apparent later in life.

CLINICAL FINDINGS

Nevus sebaceus is a unilateral, circumscribed, raised, usually solitary, yellow or yellow–brown, hairless plaque with a smooth, velvety surface (Fig. 92.1). The lesion may be rounded, linear or irregular, and it varies in size from small papules to large areas of involvement. In rare instances, the lesions are extensive and multiple. The most common sites are the scalp, the face, the forehead and the cheeks, but lesions may be located elsewhere. Nevus sebaceus may enlarge gradually.

Associations

The association of extensive sebaceus nevi with other conditions such as epilepsy, mental retardation, neurological defects, and skeletal deformities is known as 'nevus sebaceus syndrome' (Fig. 92.2).

Complications

After puberty, various secondary neoplasms develop secondarily within nevus sebaceus in about 10% of patients. Most of these lesions are trichoblastomas (Fig. 92.3) (which in the past were considered basal cell epitheliomas) or syringocystadenoma papilliferum. Less common are nodular hidradenomas, syringomas, sebaceous epitheliomas, chondroid syringomas, trichilemmomas and proliferating trichilemmal cysts.

HISTOPATHOLOGICAL FINDINGS

Prepubescent lesions appear as clusters of tiny, pyriform, sebaceous lobules associated with vellus follicles, often together with follicular germ cells and papillae, usually on the scalp (Fig. 92.4).

Post-pubescent lesions appear as papillated or digitated epidermis in association with numerous large, pyriform, sebaceous lobules, follicular germ cells and papillae. These lesions are characterized by the absence, or near absence, of terminal follicles within the lesion. Again the lesions are usually on the scalp.

ETIOLOGY AND PATHOGENESIS

The cause of nevus sebaceus is not known.

MANAGEMENT

Because of the risks of malignant change, surgical excision during childhood is recommended.

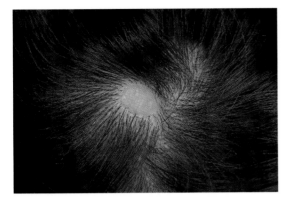

Figure 92.1
Nevus sebaceus. A well-circumscribed, raised, smooth, yellowish, alopecic plaque on the vertex of the scalp.

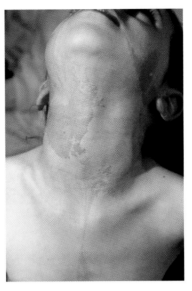

Figure 92.2
Nevus sebaceus syndrome. These large lesions are characterized by yellowish plaques composed of discrete and confluent papules. The surface of the lesion in some foci is cobblestone-like. The extensive nature of these lesions suggests they are cutaneous manifestations of other congenital vascular, skeletal or neural abnormalities, which in fact proved to be the case.

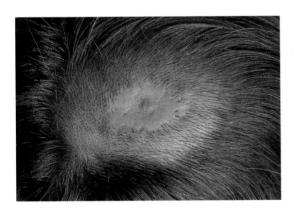

Figure 92.3
Nevus sebaceus. The blue–gray nodule that appeared at puberty within this hairless yellow plaque is a trichoblastoma. This neoplasm is frequent complication of a sebaceous nevus.

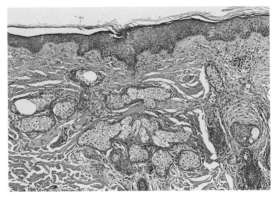

Figure 92.4
Nevus sebaceus. The diagnostic features of nevus sebaceus in this child are the cluster of sebaceous lobules in association with vellus follicles, many of these lobules are pyriform, and several structures resemble follicular germs and papillae. This lesion has a relatively flat expanse rather than the prominently papillated surface that develops at puberty. Note also that the sebaceous lobules are smaller than those in postpubescent patients.

NEVUS VERRUCOSUS

Nevus verrucosus is a localized hamartoma that is made up almost exclusively of keratinocytes.

EPIDEMIOLOGY

The lesion has been estimated to be present in 1 per 1000 live births, with equal incidence in males and females. In most cases nevus verrucosus is seen at birth but it may not be apparent until later in life.

CLINICAL FINDINGS

Nevus verrucosus consists of skin-colored or yellow–brown, keratotic papules that tend to merge to form a well-demarcated papillomatous plaque (Fig. 93.1). Their configuration is protean. Among the different shapes they assume are linear (Fig. 93.2), zosteriform (Fig. 93.3), rectangular and whorled. Such lesions often follow the Blaschko's lines and rarely cross the midline. The linear form is the commonest, especially for lesions on the limbs. When the lesions are distributed on one-half of the body, the nevus is termed nevus unius lateris. The surface of most verrucous nevi is rough and tends to become velvety and macer-ated in the folds. Lesions may gradually extend during childhood. The term 'epidermal nevus syndrome' has been given to the concurrence of an epidermal nevus and another malformation in at least one extracutaneous body system.

HISTOPATHOLOGICAL FINDINGS

Verrucous nevi may present several different histopathological patterns, of which the commonest is sharply demarcated hyperkeratosis, acanthosis and papillomatosis (Fig 93.4). In about 20% of cases, lesions assume features of epidermolytic hyperkeratosis, focal acantholytic dyskeratosis, seborrheic dermatosis and cornoid lamellation.

ETIOLOGY AND PATHOGENESIS

The cause of nevus verrucosus is unknown.

MANAGEMENT

The definitive therapy is surgical excision. Laser vaporization and dermoabrasion are alternative treatments.

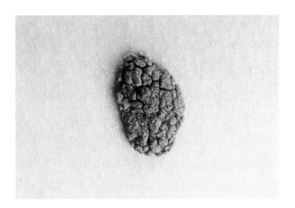

Figure 93.1
Nevus verrucosus. The lesions consist of closely set verrucous papules that coalesce to form a well-demarcated, papillomatous plaque.

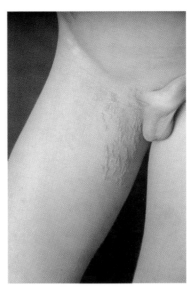

Figure 93.2
Nevus verrucosus. This unilateral lesion was present at birth and consists of pink keratotic papules, some in linear array.

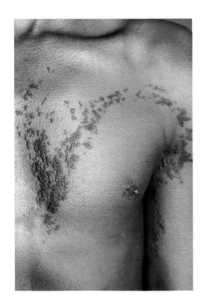

Figure 93.3
Nevus verrucosus. This unilateral nevus follows Blaschko's lines and stops sharply at the midline.

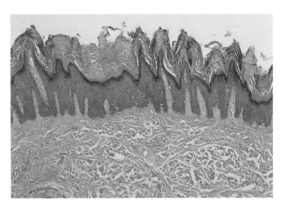

Figure 93.4
Nevus verrucosus. This epidermal nevus is characterized by a digitated thickened epidermis, hypergranulosis and a basket-woven appearance, and laminated and compact orthokeratosis.

PALMOPLANTAR HEREDITARY KERATODERMA

Palmoplantar hereditary keratodermas (PPHK) are a heterogeneous group of diseases characterized by erythema and hyperkeratosis of the palms and soles. They are distinguishable by other clinical features, associated abnormalities, and mode of inheritance. These conditions can be divided into two forms – diffuse and focal PPHK.

DIFFUSE PALMOPLANTAR HEREDITARY KERATODERMA

UNNA–THOST DISEASE

Unna–Thost disease is thought to be the most common type of PPHK. It usually manifests itself at 2–5 years of age with a diffuse erythema. Hyperkeratosis then commences at the margins of the soles and extends to the center. The disease is bilateral, symmetrical and has no tendency to spread to extensor surfaces (Figs 94.1 and 94.2). Initially, it has sharp borders surrounded by an erythematous halo. Marked hyperhidrosis is usual. Histologically, the disorder is characterized by compact hyperkeratosis, hypergranulosis and moderate acanthosis (Fig. 94.3). It is determined by an autosomal-dominant gene.

EPIDERMOLYTIC PALMOPLANTAR HEREDITARY KERATODERMA OF VORNER

Epidermolytic PPHK of Vorner may be present at birth or it may appear during the first months of life. It resembles Unna–Thost disease but hyperhidrosis is not a common finding. It is characterized by histological features of epidermolytic hyperkeratosis. The disease is inherited via an autosomal-dominant trait.

MAL DE MELEDA

Mal de Meleda is a very rare transgrediens disorder. It is a progressive form of PPHK comprising a glove and sock hyperkeratosis that does not usually have sharply defined margins. Hyperkeratotic plaques may occasionally appear, especially on the elbows and the knees. Hyperhidrosis with maceration and malodour is always present. This disease is very similar to progressive PPHK of Greither except that it is persistent and is inherited as a recessive trait. Histopathologically, mal de Meleda is characterized by epidermal hyperplasia, hyperkeratosis and inflammatory infiltrate around the dermal vessels.

PROGRESSIVE PALMOPLANTAR HEREDITARY KERATODERMA OF GREITHER

Progressive PPHK of Greither is an autosomal-dominant disorder that is characterized by diffuse keratoderma with hyperhidrosis extending to the dorsal aspect of the feet (transgrediens pattern). In addition, keratotic patches may develop on the limbs (progrediens pattern). The disease tends to improve spontaneously in middle age. It is essentially different from mal de Meleda in that it has a dominant mode of inheritance.

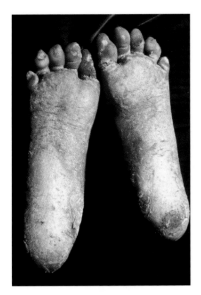

Figure 94.7
Mutilating keratoderma. The soles are covered by diffuse hyperkeratosis. Similar changes are present on the balls of the toes. Fissures have formed in hyperkeratotic zones. The process is associated with loss of digits.

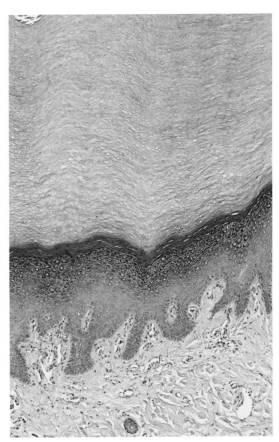

Figure 94.9
Mutilating keratoderma (Vohwinkel's disease). The granular zone is strikingly thickened and makes up almost one-half of the thickness of the viable epidermis. The configuration of the epidermis is psoriasiform. Diagnostic features of Vohwinkel's disease are that each corneocyte is punctuated by a small, round nucleus and that the parakeratotic cornified layer is associated with hyper-granulosis. No other keratoderma of the palms and soles has such an affiliation.

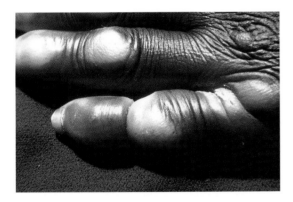

Figure 94.8
Mutilating keratoderma. Hyperkeratosis involves the dorsum of the fingers. Note also changes of pseudoainhum (i.e. focal constrictions of the digits).

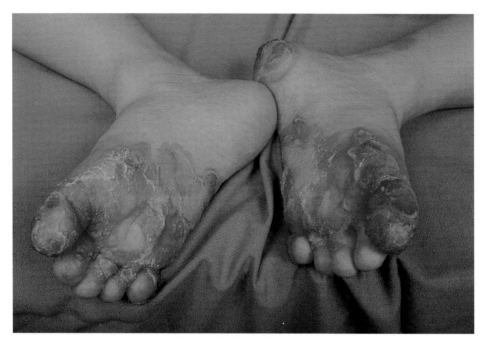

Figure 94.10
Olmsted syndrome. Progressive, well-defined painful plantar lesions can be seen.

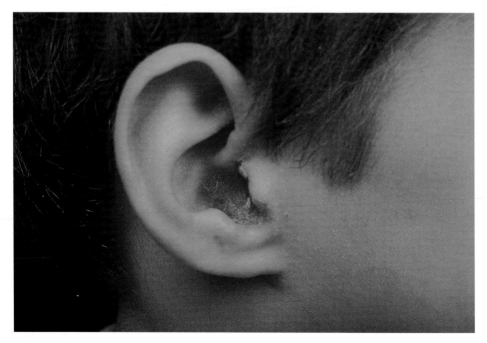

Figure 94.11
Olmsted syndrome. The perioreficial hyperkeratosis is a characteristic sign of the disease.

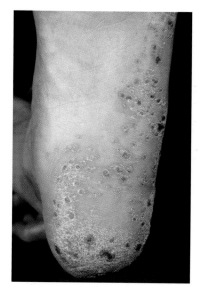

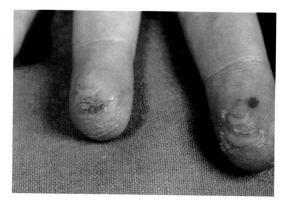

Figure 94.14
Tyrosinemia type II. Hyperkeratotic lesions tend to follow the dermatoglyphic lines and are whitish, yellowish or blackish.

Figure 94.12
Punctate keratoderma. More than one-half of the sole is involved by punctate keratotic lesions. Many of these areas are discrete and others tend to confluence. The lesions are not confined to the major skin creases, but are scattered diffusely.

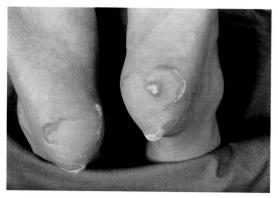

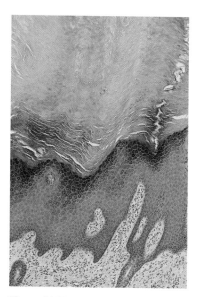

Figure 94.13
Tyrosinemia type II. Arcuate and nummular lesions are characterized by whitish and yellowish hyperkeratosis.

Figure 94.15
Palmoplantar keratoderma in tyrosinemia type II. This specimen was taken from a patient with clinically prominent hyperkeratosis. That change is reflected histopathologically in a cornified layer, thick even by standards of volar skin, slight papillation of the viable epidermis, hypergranulosis and epidermal hyperplasia.

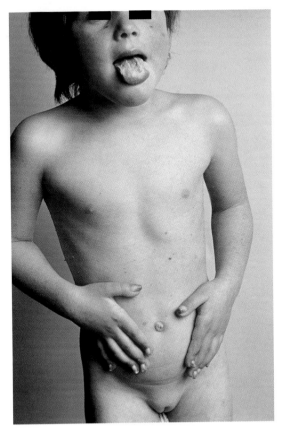

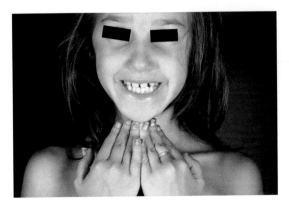

Figure 94.17
Congenital pachyonychia. Hypertrophy and distortion of nails are accompanied by hyperkeratotic changes on the lips and by dental abnormalities.

Figure 94.16
Congenital pachyonychia. The tongue is hyperkeratotic and all the nails are dystrophic.

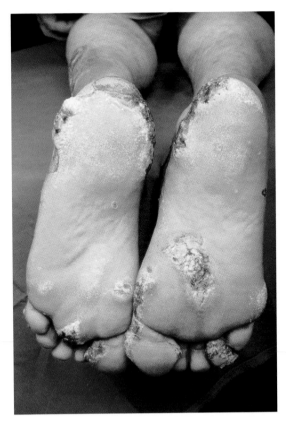

Figure 94.18
Congenital pachyonychia. Plantar keratoderma is symmetrical, non-transgrediens and mainly localized over pressure points.

95 PELLAGRA

Pellagra is a systemic disease caused by an inadequate dietary supply of nicotinic acid (niacin) and nicotinamide. These two substances are called pellagra-preventing factors, from which the term 'vitamin PP' is derived. The disease is characterized by the classic triad of dermatitis, diarrhea and dementia – the three Ds. Pellagra still exists in developing countries, affecting children and adults, whereas in the Western world the disease is rare and is observed almost exclusively in patients affected by chronic alcohol abuse, gastrointestinal diseases or severe psychiatric disturbances.

CLINICAL FINDINGS

Pellagra begins on sun-exposed areas, such as the face and the dorsum of the hands. It consists of erythema and scaling, sometimes accompanied by pruritus. The skin is smooth and edematous; vesicles and blisters may appear, with fissures and scales (Fig. 95.1). Scaly desquamation can be followed by wizened and glazed skin (Fig. 95.2). On the face, erythema predominates on the nose and cheeks, giving a symmetric 'butterfly' eruption (see Fig. 95.2). A well-marginated eruption, Casal's necklace, can be seen on the neck, closing in the back and going down to the sternal area. The erythema fades in winter and recurs in spring. With time, the skin becomes rougher, drier, and pigmented with a darker margin. The lips are dry and fissured (see Fig. 95.2). The oral mucosa is red, dry and smooth, with numerous aphthous lesions, which may be large. The tongue is usually swollen and magenta in color, but it can also be atrophic and black. Vulvar involvement is less common. The diaper area is particularly affected in infants.

Diarrhea is one of the symptoms that marks the severity of the disease. Feces are frequent, water-like at the beginning and then with a bloody aspect. Neurological signs consist of weakness, insomnia, and mental depression. Without significant improvement in the diet, the course is chronic.

LABORATORY FINDINGS

The mean serum values for serotonin and its metabolite 5-hydroxyindoleacetic acid (5–HIAA) are significantly higher in pellagra patients than in the general population.

HISTOPATHOLOGICAL FINDINGS

Evolving lesions are characterized by pallid, ballooned keratinocytes in the spinous and granular layers (Fig. 95.3) and foci of parakeratosis that contain neutrophils.

MANAGEMENT

The administration of oral nicotinamide at a dose of 100–500 mg/day is rapidly effective. Severe cases necessitate intravenous treatment. A protein-rich diet is highly recommended for all patients.

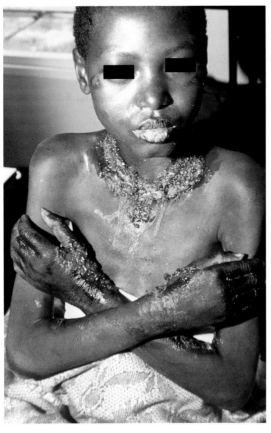

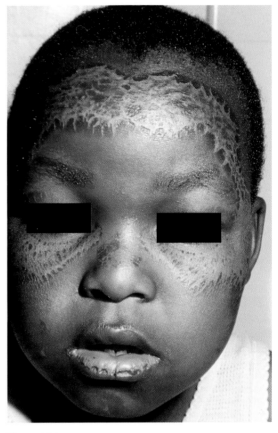

Figure 95.1
Pellagra. Acute changes (ulcerations and vegetations) involve the lips, the upper part of the chest and the hands. Post-inflammatory hyperpigmentation is also evident in these areas.

Figure 95.2
Pellagra. Ichthyosiform hyperpigmented plaques are present on the forehead, the nose and the intraorbital regions, giving a mask-like appearance. The lips are also affected by the process.

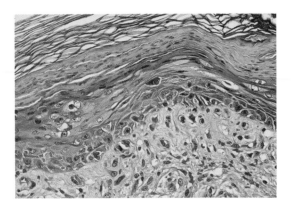

Figure 95.3
Pellagra. Note the confluent necrosis of the epidermis beneath a normal basket-woven cornified layer; the pallor of the granular and spinous zones; the focal thinning of the epidermis; and the sparse, perivascular lymphocytic infiltrate. These features are also manifestations of acrodermatitis enteropathica and necrolytic migratory erythema.

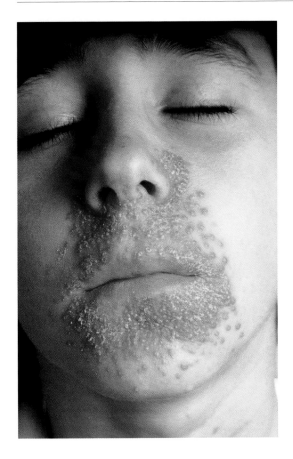

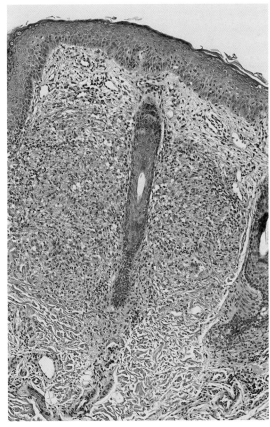

Figure 97.1
Perioral dermatitis. Scaly and crusted, reddish papules are present around the mouth and the lower portion of the nose.

Figure 97.2
Perioral dermatitis. This papular lesion is characterized by granulomatous perifollicutis together with lymphoplasmacytic infiltrates.

PILOMATRICOMA

Pilomatricoma is a benign adnexal tumor composed of cells resembling those of the hair matrix.

EPIDEMIOLOGY

Forty per cent of pilomatricomas begin before the age of 10 years, and more than 60% manifest themselves before the age of 20 years with a peak between 8 and 13 years of age.

Pilomatricomas represent 10% of nodules and tumors in children 16 years of age and younger. The neoplasm is more common in females than in males.

CLINICAL FINDINGS

Pilomatricomas typically manifest as solitary, irregularly shaped papules, nodules or tumors. Early lesions are cystic (Fig. 98.1), whereas more advanced lesions may develop flattened, polygonal outlines (the so-called 'tent sign') and are rock hard. In most instances, the epidermis is unaffected. Pilomatricomas often assume a blue or grayish hue, although shades of red and yellow, as well as normal skin tone, are also seen. In some certain fully developed lesions, chalk-white concretions (calcified or ossified foci) may be discerned within the nodule (Fig. 98.2). Affected people are often asymptomatic, although about 50% of patients report some tenderness when the lesion is palpated. Most pilomatricomas enlarge slowly over several months. Once the lesion has calcified, there is no tendency for regression. In about 70% of patients, lesions arise on the head (see Figs 98.1 and 98.2) (particularly the face) and the neck; other lesions are situated, in decreasing frequency, on the arms, the thighs and the trunk. The palms, the soles and the mucous membranes have not been reported to be involved to date.

Carcinomatous transformation, although rare, has been reported in pediatric patients.

Associations

Patients with myotonic dystrophy have a higher incidence of pilomatricoma than the general population.

LABORATORY FINDINGS

Radiographic examination demonstrates the presence of calcium salts. Calcification is common in pilomatricoma, occurring in about 80% of all cases.

HISTOPATHOLOGICAL FINDINGS

In the early stage pilomatricoma is characterized by a cystic structure that is lined by infundibular and matrical epithelium and that contains cornified cells, which may be 'shadow cells'. The shadow cells exhibit pale, eosinophilic ghosts of nuclei (Figs 98.3 and 98.4). These cells undergo progressive calcification. Subsequent ossification of shadow cells occurs as a consequence of metaplasia of fibrocytes and osteoblasts.

ETIOLOGY AND PATHOGENESIS

It is not known whether this tumor is derived directly from the hair matrix cells or from pluripotential cutaneous epithelial stem cells.

MANAGEMENT

Complete but conservative excision is curative.

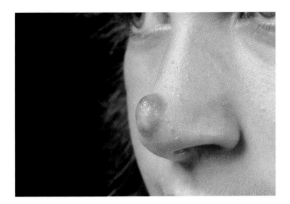

Figure 98.1
Pilomatricoma. The tumor is firm and yellow–brown, with whitish areas where the calcification is more superficial.

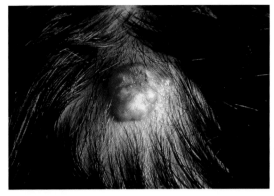

Figure 98.2
Giant pilomatricoma. This multilobulated nodule is ulcerated and crusted. Whitish zones at the periphery represent areas of calcification.

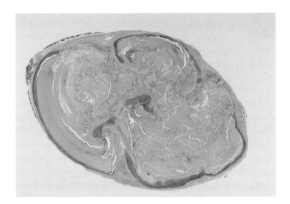

Figure 98.3

Figures 98.3 and 98.4
Pilomatricoma. Cystic stage (Fig. 98.3) – even a large lesion may be mostly cystic. The lining of the cyst consists entirely of matrical cells. As these cells mature, they become cornified in a faulty attempt to form hair shafts. Those cells demonstrate karyolysis; ghosts of nuclei have prompted the designation shadow cell (Fig. 98.4).

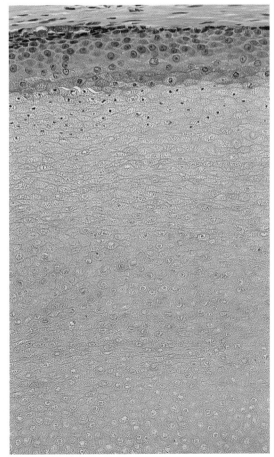

Figure 98.4

Pityriasis lichenoides, also known as guttate parapsoriasis, is a self-limited, polymorphous skin disorder of unknown origin. It is characterized by erythematous papules that tend to evolve into scales, vesicles, pustules and crusts, sometimes with central necrosis. The disease is usually divided into an acute form (acute guttate parapsoriasis, parapsoriasis varioliformis, Mucha–Habermann disease, pityriasis lichenoides et varioliformis acuta) and a chronic form (pityriasis lichenoides chronica, guttate parapsoriasis of Juliusberg). A new classification based on the distribution of the lesions subdivides the disease into three forms – diffuse, central and peripheral.

EPIDEMIOLOGY

Pytiriasis lichenoides is an uncommon disorder that affects males and females with equal frequency. In about 20% of patients, it begins in childhood. The age distribution curve show two peaks, one at 5 years and one at 10 years.

CLINICAL FINDINGS

The acute form of pityriasis lichenoides is characterized by pink, orange or purpuric papules that may evolve into vesicles that resolve with hemorrhagic crusts (Figs 99.1 and 99.2). Some papules and vesicles ulcerate and heal to leave varioliform scars. The lesions tend to be numerous and to erupt in crops, and they are accompanied by fever and malaise in some patients. The course of the disease runs from a few weeks to several months.

In the chronic form (Figs 99.3 and 99.4) the lesions consist of reddish-brown papules with an adherent central scale that tends to separate spontaneously. The lesions clear without scarring, leaving only transient skin discolorations. The disease course may be as long as a few years.

Both forms of pityriasis lichenoides are asymptomatic or accompanied by slight itching. Because both types of lesions often coexist in the same patient and no correlation seems to exist between the severity of the skin lesions and the overall duration of the disease, a classification based on the distribution of the lesions has been proposed. The diffuse form, which is the most common, is characterized by acute and chronic lesions scattered over the entire body surface, except the palms, the soles, and the mucosae. The central form usually involves the trunk, whereas the less common peripheral form is limited to the limbs and buttocks and tends to last longer.

HISTOPATHOLOGICAL FINDINGS

Stereotypical changes of the lesions of pityriasis lichenoides are a wedge-shaped, superficial and deep, perivascular lymphocytic infiltrate; edema of the papillary dermis; extravasated erythrocytes in the papillary dermis and sometimes in the epidermis; lymphocytes aligned along the dermoepidermal junction together with vacuolar alteration; and necrotic keratinocytes disposed as solitary units in the lower half of the epidermis (Figs 99.5 and 99.6).

ETIOLOGY AND PATHOGENESIS

The etiopathogenesis of pityriasis lichenoides remains obscure.

MANAGEMENT

Topical treatment with cortisone, tars, salicylate creams and various vitamin ointments have been used as symptomatic therapy with modest improvement. Long-term treatment with oral erythromycin has been proposed, but further confirmation is needed. Ultraviolet-B irradiation seems to be effective in alleviating symptoms without major side effects.

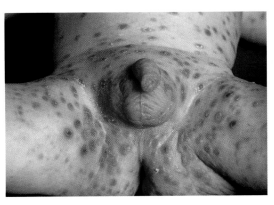

Figure 99.2
Acute pityriasis lichenoides (diffuse form). Pink macules, reddish papules and ulcerated papules covered by scaly crust are widespread. Note also the confluence of some papules to form plaques.

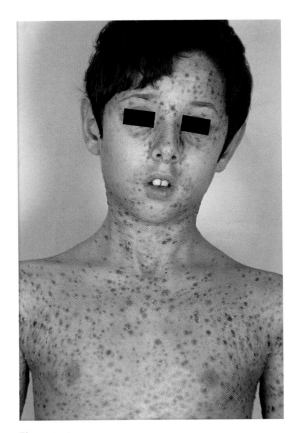

Figure 99.1
Acute pityriasis lichenoides (diffuse form). Purpuric macules, papules, and hemorrhagic, crusted papules involve the face, the neck, the trunk and the extremities.

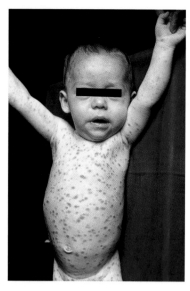

Figure 99.3
Chronic pityriasis lichenoides (diffuse form). Rust-brown macules and papules cover the trunk and extremities.

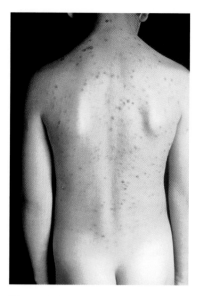

Figure 99.4
Chronic pityriasis lichenoides (central form). Reddish-brown and scaly papules are seen on the trunk, but few are seen on the extremities.

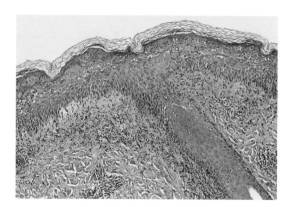

Figure 99.3

Figure 99.5 and 99.6
Acute pityriasis lichenoides. This lesion of Mucha–Habermann disease is of recent onset because the cornified layer is almost entirely of basket-weave design and parakeratotic cells have not yet emerged. The process is that of Mucha–Habermann disease because the infiltrate of lymphocytes is wedge-shaped, perivascular and interstitial, and because the infiltrate obscures the dermoepidermal junction focally. Within the epidermis are signs of spongiosis and ballooning as well as hints of scaly crusts.

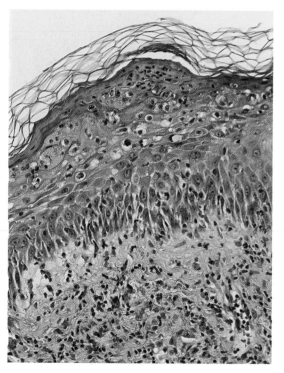

Figure 99.4

Pityriasis rosea is an acute, common, self-limited inflammatory disease of unknown cause characterized by a distinctive eruption.

EPIDEMIOLOGY

Pityriasis rosea is common during adolescence. Only 5% of patients are less than 5 years of age. It affects males and females equally. Seasonal incidence appears to vary according to geographical location. In temperate climates, it is more frequent in the spring.

CLINICAL FINDINGS

In about 80% of cases, the disease starts with a single isolated lesion, called the herald patch, which may appear anywhere on the body. This initial lesion is a round or oval, sharply defined plaque with a pink center and a slightly elevated and finely scaled border. It is 20–60 mm in diameter. After a few days or weeks, secondary lesions (Fig. 100.1) appear, usually on the trunk, the neck and the proximal parts of the extremities. These lesions are smaller, pink or light brown, with a center that has an appearance of cigarette paper, surrounded by a typical collar of scales.

Particularly in children, pityriasis rosea may be atypical in its morphology and distribution. Various types of lesions have been described in atypical variants, especially during the early stages of the eruption, as vesicular, urticarial, papular purpuric, and erythema multiforme-like. Pityriasis rosea may be unilateral and may occur on the face, the extremities and the oral mucous membranes. Subjective symptoms are usually absent or consist of slight pruritus. One-fifth of patients have had acute infections before the appearance of the disease. Spontaneous resolution generally occurs within 4–12 weeks.

HISTOPATHOLOGICAL FINDINGS

A superficial perivascular, predominantly lymphocytic infiltrate is associated with slight edema of the papillary dermis and extravasated erythrocytes, both in the papillary dermis and within the epidermis. Focal spongiosis, slight epidermal hyperplasia and mounds of parakeratosis are also seen (Fig. 100.2).

ETIOLOGY AND PATHOGENESIS

The etiology of pityriasis rosea is unknown. Many conditions have been suggested as possible causes or precipitating factors – viral or bacterial infections, the atopic state and seborrheic dermatitis.

MANAGEMENT

No treatment is required. If itching is present, a mild corticosteroid cream may be useful.

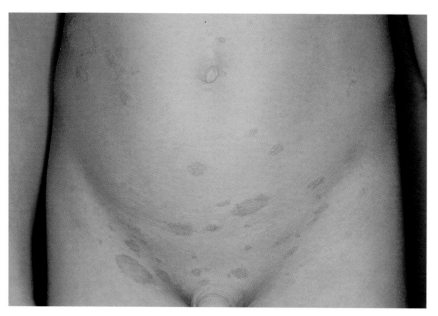

Figure 100.1
Pityriasis rosea. Oval papules and plaques have reddish-brown scales, mostly at their periphery.

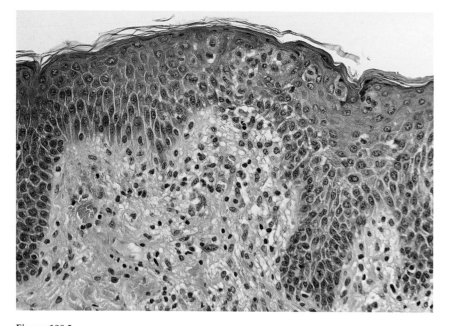

Figure 100.2
Pityriasis rosea. This lesion is in its early stages because of the absence of mounds of parakeratosis. The superficial perivascular lymphocytic infiltrate, the slight epidermal hyperplasia, the slight edema of the papillary dermis with extravasated erythrocytesm and the slight focal spongiosis are characteristic of this condition.

PITYRIASIS ROTUNDA

Pityriasis rotunda is an unusual disorder of keratinization characterized by persistent, round or oval, sharply demarcated, scaling patches, which are either darker or lighter than the surrounding skin.

EPIDEMIOLOGY

Although pityriasis rotunda may begin in infancy or childhood, the majority of patients who have been reported on have been 20–45 years of age. The condition has been described most often in Japanese people and in South African and West Indian blacks. In Italy, pityriasis rotunda is common among Sardinian people.

CLINICAL FINDINGS

Pityriasis rotunda is characterized by strikingly circular or occasionally oval, hypopigmented or hyperpigmented patches (Fig. 101.1) covered with fine scales. The edges of the patches are sharply demarcated from normal skin, and there is no evidence of inflammation. Lesions vary in size from 5 to 280 mm in diameter, and they may be numerous (as many as 30) and become confluent. Sites of predilection are the trunk and the limbs. The lesions are asymptomatic. The condition tend to be chronic.

HISTOPATHOLGICAL FINDINGS

Histological sections of pityriasis rotunda show laminated orthokeratosis, thinning of the granular layer and hyperpigmentation of the basal keratinocytes (Fig. 101.2), accompanied by a sparse superficial lymphohistiocytic infiltrate.

ETIOLOGY AND PATHOGENESIS

The etiopathogenesis is unknown. The clinical and microscopic features suggest that pityriasis rotunda is a special localized variant of acquired ichthyosis.

MANAGEMENT

Treatment with topical 'keratolytic' agents may ameliorate the condition.

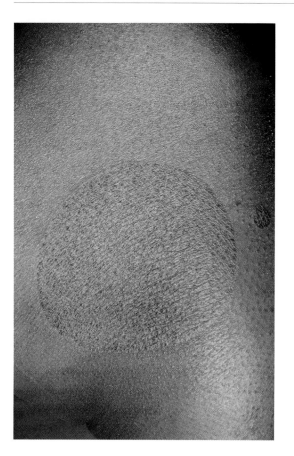

Figure 101.1
Pityriasis rotunda. This large nummular patch is markedly hyperpigmented and is covered by subtle scales.

Figure 101.2
Pityriasis rotunda. Histopathological features of pityriasis rotunda are basket-woven and laminar orthokeratosis together with a thin granular layer and hyperpigmentation of the basal keratinocytes.

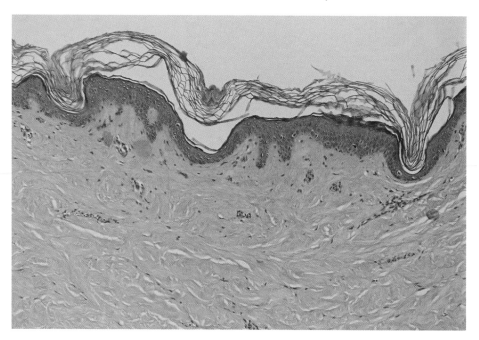

PITYRIASIS RUBRA PILARIS

Pityriasis rubra pilaris is a benign, erythematous, squamous disorder. It is characterized by follicular plugging, perifollicular erythema, a cephalic rash and palmoplantar hyperkeratosis. It affects prepubertal children and young adults more commonly than others.

EPIDEMIOLOGY

Pityriasis rubra pilaris is a rare disorder. It occurs in one case in every 3500 new patients. Males and females are affected with equal frequency. In childhood there is a peak age of onset between 3 years and 6 years.

CLINICAL FINDINGS

The most characteristic clinical feature is a follicular verrucous papule, about 1 mm in diameter, with a central keratotic plug. This papule is surrounded by a classic yellow–orange ring. Initially these papules are discrete, but they soon coalesce to form hyperkeratotic plaques (Figs 102.1 and 102.2) that have a characteristic 'pachydermic' appearance with an exaggerated furrowing of the skin. In children, the elbows and the knees (see Fig. 102.2) are frequently affected, followed by, in decreasing order of frequency, the dorsal aspect of the feet and hands (Fig. 102.3) and the ankles; the involvement of the dorsal aspect of the proximal phalanges (see Fig. 102.3) is not as common as it is in adults.

The second important diagnostic element is a palmoplantar keratoderma, which is present in most cases. It can be distinguished from ichthyotic keratoderma by its salmon color and by the presence of edema that can sometimes be partially disabling. The dermatitis has a sharply demarcated border that is usually delimited by the dorsal aspect of the limbs. The Achilles tendon is frequently involved.

The third diagnostic element is a cephalic rash (see Fig. 102.1), which sometimes extends beyond the neck in a cape-like formation; again, this rash has sharp borders.

The unifying element of all lesions is their characteristic salmon color, which is therefore of particular diagnostic importance. Pruritus can occur but is usually mild. In a few cases there is a burning sensation. The disease usually resolves spontaneously after a variable period of time ranging from a few months to several years.

HISTOPATHOLOGICAL FINDINGS

The crucial findings are in the stratum corneum, where squares of orthokeratosis and parakeratosis alternate in chess board fashion (Fig. 102.4). Follicular plugging is not required to make the diagnosis of pityriasis rubra pilaris; in fact, in certain anatomic sites, such as the palms and the soles, the ostia of adnexal structures are not plugged.

ETIOLOGY AND PATHOGENESIS

Although a viral cause can be postulated by the fact that a febrile illness precedes the onset of pityriasis rubra pilaris in many cases, no specific etiology has been demonstrated.

Some papers claim a possible role for a serine protein, retinol binding protein, in the development of the disease.

MANAGEMENT

Topical treatment with cortisone, tars, salicylate creams and vitamin A have been used as symptomatic therapy with modest improvement. Synthetic retinoids such as isotretinoin and etretinate have also been used and seem to influence the course of pityriasis rubra pilaris positively even though the response to this treatment still remains unpredictable. Stanazolol has also been used, with inconstant results.

Phototherapy in its various forms is of little help in pityriasis rubra pilaris.

abnormal elastic tissue, whereas in late lesions elastic fibers are completely obscured by abundant deposits of calcium. The appearance of the abnormal elastic tissue has been compared to steel wool and balls of yarn.

ETIOLOGY AND PATHOGENESIS

Pseudoxanthoma elasticum is a clinically and genetically heterogeneous disease. At least two autosomal-dominant and three autosomal-recessive subtypes have been recognized. These subtypes differ in the severity of the ophthalmological and vascular manifestations. The autosomal-recessive forms are the commoner types. The basic defect of pseudo-

xanthoma elasticum remains unknown. It is unclear whether the deposition of calcium is a primary or a secondary event.

MANAGEMENT

The appearance of the skin of patients with pseudoxanthoma elasticum may be improved by plastic surgery. Periodic cardiovascular surveillance is absolutely necessary. Smoking should be discouraged. The usefulness of reducing calcium intake is debated, but it seems a reasonable measure. Ophthalmological examination should be undertaken annually. Laser photocoagulation is a procedure of great benefit in preventing retinal hemorrhage. Genetic counselling should be offered.

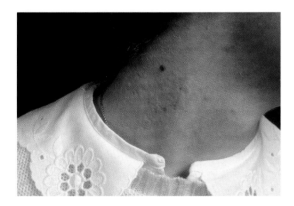

Figure 108.1
Pseudoxanthoma elasticum. Yellowish and xanthoma-like papules are confluent in plaques, giving the affected area a 'pricked-chicken-skin' appearance. The sides of the neck are a site of predilection.

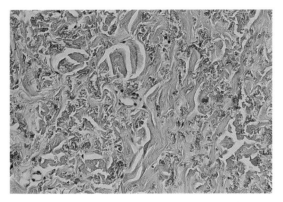

Figure 108.2
Pseudoxanthoma elasticum. In the reticular dermis, the distinctive finding is accumulation of irregularly clumped basophilic elastic fibers whose appearance resembles steel wool or balls of yarn. Abnormal elastic fibers are demonstrated vividly by orcein stain.

PSORIASIS

Psoriasis is a common chronic skin disease characterized by sharply demarcated erythematous scaling lesions that especially involve the scalp and the extensor surfaces in adolescents and adults, and the scalp and the skin folds in infants.

EPIDEMIOLOGY

The prevalence of psoriasis differs greatly from country to country. Available findings show a range between 0 and 5% in the general population. Psoriasis in childhood is not so common as in adults, but there are no definitive epidemiological studies. Psoriasis seems to have earlier onset in females than in males.

CLINICAL FINDINGS

Many clinical forms of psoriasis may occur in children. Guttate psoriasis is the commonest form of psoriasis in children. It is characterized by a sudden appearance, usually after an upper respiratory tract infection of streptococcal origin. Drop-like, round or oval lesions are scattered over the body, sparing the face (Fig. 109.1). The eruption is asymptomatic and lasts for several weeks, showing the tendency to heal spontaneously, at least in part.

Nummular psoriasis is less common in children than in adults but it presents the same clinical features. Sharply demarcated erythematous scaling lesions (Fig. 109.2) are usually located on the elbows, the knees, the scalp and the lumbosacral areas. The diaper area is involved in almost all infants. Not infrequently in children the disease involves the folds (inverse psoriasis), the genitalia, the eyelids and the palms and the soles. Large plaques may form by coalescence of several lesions. An isomorphic response (the Koebner phenomenon) may appear at sites of trauma.

Erythrodermic psoriasis arising *de novo* is occasionally observed in the neonatal period. Generalization of pre-existing cutaneous lesions (Fig. 109.3) may occur in association with drug allergy, atopic dermatitis, sunburn and leukemia.

Pustular psoriasis in children is rare and presents in three main clinical forms. The generalized form (von Zumbush variety) is characterized by an explosive, diffuse eruption of sterile, pinhead pustules associated with high fever, malaise, anorexia and pain (Fig. 109.4). This form is not usually preceded by psoriasis vulgaris. The annular form is commoner and less severe; it is characterized by erythema and pustules in circinate patterns.

The localized palmoplantar form (Barber variety) is characterized by recurrent crops of pustules of 2–4 mm in diameter within areas of erythema and scaling.

The course of psoriasis is usually chronic with remissions and exacerbations. Seasonal variations are common. Erythrodermic and pustular psoriasis appear to be less severe in children than in adults.

Associations

In all of the juvenile forms of psoriasis, the involvement of nails is rather common (seen in about 50% of patients). Involved nails display pitting, discoloration, onycholysis and subungueal hyperkeratosis. Whereas psoriatic

HISTOPATHOLOGICAL FINDINGS

Bullous impetigo

The dominant change in bullous impetigo is a blister situated in the uppermost part of the spinous zone, the granular zone, or the subcorneal zone. Within the blister, a few acantholytic cells and neutrophils are usually apparent (Fig. 112.7). Only a sparse infiltrate of lymphocytes and neutrophils is seen around the vessels of the superficial plexus.

Non-bullous impetigo

A discrete collection of neutrophils is housed beneath the stratum corneum in the upper part of the spinous zone and in the granular zone. There may be slight edema of the papillary dermis and a sparse superficial perivascular and interstitial infiltrate of lymphocytes and neutrophils (Fig. 112.8).

ETIOLOGY AND PATHOGENESIS

Impetigo contagiosa and the other skin diseases dealt with in this chapter are caused by bacteria. The commonest cause of non-bullous impetigo contagiosa is group A beta-hemolytic streptococci. *Staphylococcus aureus* is the major cause of bullous impetigo. In impetigo contagiosa caused by streptococci and staphylococci, the bacteria produce toxins, which are responsible for the clinical features of the disease, in that they function as exfoliatin, causing keratinocytes to separate from one another (acantholysis) at the level of the granular layer.

MANAGEMENT

Localized impetigo contagiosa may respond to topical antibiotics such as mupirocin (pseudomonic acid), bacitracin ointment or erythromycin. In addition to the topical treatment, it is always advisable to give a systemic antibiotic, although it is questionable whether this prevents the rare poststreptococcal glomerulonephritis. If streptococci are known to be the etiological agent, then oral penicillin or erythromycin is curative. When a specific bacterial cause is not known, or if lesions are bullous, then oral therapy with erythromycin, cephalosporins, dicloxacillin, or other antibiotics with effective antistaphylococcal activity should be given.

SCALDED SKIN STAPHYLOCOCCAL SYNDROME

Scalded skin staphylococcal syndrome is a rare, extensive, exfoliative form of pyogenic skin infection produced by *Staphylococcus aureus*. The onset is under 5 years of age; the median age at onset is 2 years.

CLINICAL FINDINGS

Clinically, the disease starts during or after a rhinitis, a conjunctivitis or a purulent otitis. It begins with a scarlatiniform erythema, accompanied by cutaneous tenderness (Fig. 112.3). It involves folds and periorificial regions. The toxic syndrome is characterized by high fever, malaise and vomiting. Within 24–48 hours the disease usually progresses from the scarlatiniform eruption to wrinkling with large, flaccid blisters. The Nicholsky sign is positive, even in apparently uninvolved skin. The rupture of the roofs of blisters causes large erosions that are red, wet and bordered by remnants of the roofs of blisters (see Fig. 112.3). The skin looks scalded. Severe mucosal involvement does not usually occur. If antibiotic therapy is given quickly, rapid post-inflammatory desquamation occurs, with complete restitution of epithelium. Recovery is the rule and occurs in 6–12 years.

Complications

Complications of scalded skin staphylococcal syndrome are the same as those of an extensive burn, as well as sepsis, pneumonia or other internal localizations.

LABORATORY FINDINGS

In scalded skin staphylococcal syndrome, the white blood cell count is augmented and the erythrocyte sedimentation rate is elevated. *Staphylococcus aureus* may be isolated from the exudate.

HISTOPATHOLOGICAL FINDINGS

There are sparse, superficial, perivascular mixed cell infiltrates of neutrophils and lymphocytes, subcorneal pustules that contain variable numbers of acantholytic cells, and epidermal necrosis in varying degree.

ETIOLOGY AND PATHOGENESIS

The syndrome is caused by an exotoxin produced by staphylococci of phage group 2. The exotoxin cleaves the epidermis beneath the stratum granulosum.

MANAGEMENT

Treatment consists of isolation of the patient, administration of penicillinase-resistant penicillin analogs, local disinfection with silver nitrate (1:1000 aqueous) or potassium permanganate solution, and restoration of the electrolyte balance.

FURUNCLES

Furuncles, also known as boils, are acute, deep-seated perifollicular abscesses caused by bacteria. They are not usually seen in infants and are commonest in the postpubertal period and in later childhood.

CLINICAL FINDINGS

Furuncles are tender and painful, red nodules, which may become fluctuant and enlarge to about 10 mm or more in diameter. From the nodules, purulent blood-tinged material may discharge (Fig. 112.4). The confluence of many furuncles is called a carbuncle. Furuncles typically heal with hyperpigmentation, and some of them may scar. They may be recurrent.

HISTOPATHOLOGICAL FINDINGS

Histopathologically, neutrophils not only clog widely dilated infundibula, they are present within walls of infundibula and in the periinfundibular dermis together with lymphocytes and a variable number of histiocytes. In furuncles, the suppuration always spreads along the lower segment of follicles as well as the upper segment. Gram staining may reveal bacteria within the cytoplasm of some neutrophils. A carbuncle develops when suppuration involves the infundibula of adjacent follicles and also extends far down along the inferior segments of a follicle to the level of the deep reticular dermis or the subcutaneous fat (Fig. 112.9).

ETIOLOGY AND PATHOGENESIS

The most important etiological agent is *Staphylococcus aureus*, but the strains differ from those of impetigo (e.g. a different range of groups, including phage type 80/81). The pathogenesis of furuncles is thought to be the production of factors that attract polymorphonuclear leukocytes and determine whether a particular strain of *Staphylococcus aureus* will elicit an inflammatory response on invasion of the hair follicle.

MANAGEMENT

Furuncles respond well to topical antibacterial treatment. Incision and drainage are indicated, too.

ECTHYMA

Ecthyma is a rare, deeper form of bacterial infection of the skin.

CLINICAL FINDINGS

Ecthyma is characterized by an initial vesicle or pustule on an erythematous base, most often located on the buttocks and lower extremities, which is followed by the development of induration and ulceration. The ulcers may be topped by a thick, circular, adherent crust (Fig. 112.5). The lesions of ecthyma may be painful, unlike those of impetigo contagiosa, and lymphadenopathy may be present. Pigmentary changes are common on healing of ecthyma, and scars may sometimes remain.

HISTOPATHOLOGICAL FINDINGS

Ecthyma is characterized by a superficial ulcer beneath which there is a dense inflltrate of neutrophils that may extend to the upper part of the reticular dermis.

ETIOLOGY AND PATHOGENESIS

Group A beta-hemolytic streptococci are the most frequent cause of ecthyma. Poor living conditions and poor hygiene are predisposing factors.

MANAGEMENT

The disease responds well to topical and systemic treatment with antibiotics with effective antistaphylococcal activity, such as erythromycin, dicloxacillin or benzathine penicillin.

ERYSIPELA

Erysipela (streptococcal cellulitis) is rarely seen in children. It is caused by group A beta-hemolytic streptococci.

CLINICAL FINDINGS

Erysipela is characterized by a superficial, acute, well-demarcated inflammation. In newborns, it lacks the typical border and the commonest localization is the periumbilical area, but the face may also be involved. In children, the lower extremities may be involved and may have superficial bullae. In a few cases, perianal and even genital streptococcal cellulitis (dermatitis) (Fig. 112.6) has been reported, which is accompanied by painful defecation and secondary constipation, rectal bleeding and brown mucoid discharge. Systemic signs and symptoms, such as fever, chills and prostration, may be present and variably severe. Recurrences are common.

HISTOPATHOLOGICAL FINDINGS

Erysipela is characterized by sparse perivascular and interstitial infiltrate composed mostly of neutrophils, extravasation of erythrocytes and edema of the papillary dermis.

MANAGEMENT

Treatment includes topical and oral antibacterial drugs, mainly penicillin, to be continued for at least 2 weeks.

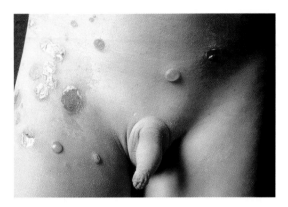

Figure 112.1
Bullous impetigo. The tense blisters rupture to leave erosions that soon are covered by scaly crusts.

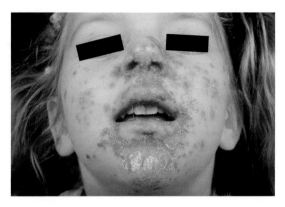

Figure 112.2
Non-bullous impetigo. The face is a site of predilection, especially around the mouth and nasal orifices. Lesions are characteristically covered by soft crusts that are the color of honey.

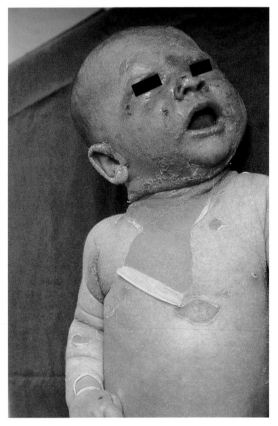

Figure 112.3
Staphylococcal scalded skin syndrome. This condition resembles scalded skin because the epidermis is gray as a consequence of necrosis and the skin is diffusely blistered.

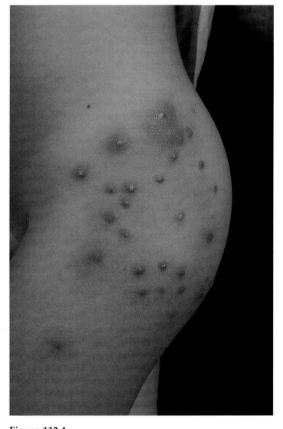

Figure 112.4
Furuncles. Typical nodulopustular lesions surrounded by an erythematous halo.

RETICULOHISTIOCYTOSIS

Reticulohistiocytosis of the skin covers a spectrum of rare clinical entities ranging from the solitary cutaneous form through the diffuse cutaneous form without systemic involvement to multicentric reticulohistiocytosis with systemic involvement. The skin lesions of all these conditions demonstrate an identical histological pattern that is characterized by the presence of numerous mononucleated or multinucleated histiocytes with abundant, eosinophilic, homogeneous to finely granular cytoplasm with a ground-glass appearance.

EPIDEMIOLOGY

All the variants of reticulohistiocytosis are extremely rare in children. Pediatric cases have been observed in patients aged from 6 to 13 years.

CLINICAL FINDINGS

Solitary cutaneous reticulohistiocytosis (reticulohistiocytoma cutis) is characterized by a single, firm, rapidly growing nodule that varies in color from yellow–brown to dark red (Fig. 114.1). This tumor most commonly involves the head and the neck, but it may be found on almost any cutaneous site. The lesion, which is often clinically misdiagnosed, occurs without evidence of systemic involvement. The onset may be preceded by a trauma and the lesion is usually self-healing in few years.

Diffuse cutaneous reticulohistiocytosis is a purely cutaneous form characterized by the eruption of firm, smooth, asymptomatic papules and nodules scattered diffusely on the skin. The color of new lesions is pink–yellow, while the older lesions show a red–brown color (Fig. 114.2). Joint or visceral lesions are absent. The lesions may involute spontaneously, but it is possible that they represent an early stage of multicentric reticulohistiocytosis before the appearance of joint and visceral manifestations.

Multicentric reticulohistiocytosis exclusively involves adults over 40 years of age and is always associated with a severe polyarthritis, which may precede the cutaneous eruption. The skin lesions are papulonodular, ranging in diameter from a few millimeters to 20 mm; they are round, translucent, and yellow–rose or yellow–brown in color. They do not tend to ulcerate and preferentially affect the fingers, the palms and the backs of the hands, the juxta-articular regions of the limbs and the face. Oral, nasal, and pharyngeal mucosa are involved in 50% of cases. Osteoarticular manifestations symmetrically involve the hands (in 80% of patients), knees (in 70%), and wrists (in 65%). There is no parallelism between the mucocutaneous and articular courses. The mucocutaneous lesions have a highly variable course and may remit spontaneously. The osteoarticular manifestations in half of the patients become stable; in the other half there is a progressive destructive course. Fever, weight loss and weakness may be present. The term 'lipoid dermatoarthritis' indicates a particular form of multicentric reticulohistiocytosis that is characterized by familial occurrence, ocular involvement (glaucoma, uveitis and cataract) and xanthomatous lesions.

Associations

In adults there is an association with an internal malignancy in 15–20% of cases. Solid tumors are the most common type of malignancy. Reticulohistiocytosis may occasionally occur in association with autoimmune diseases, systemic vasculitis and thyroid diseases.

HISTOPATHOLOGICAL FINDINGS

The histopathological findings in the three types of reticulohistiocytosis and in the various involved tissues are identical. The lesions of reticulohistiocytosis usually present as dome-shaped papules or nodules characterized by a dense diffuse infiltrate that is composed mostly of mononuclear, binucleate and multinucleate histiocytes (Figs 114.3 and 114.4). The histiocytes have a distinctive appearance, with roundish nuclei, abundant amphophilic cytoplasm, a finely granular, dark eosinophilic center and a light eosinophilic periphery ('ground-glass' cytoplasm). The number of giant cells may vary and the nuclei may be arranged haphazardly or they may align along the periphery or cluster in the center. In addition to the predominant infiltration of histiocytes, the lesions may be sprinkled with lymphocytes, eosinophils and, sometimes, neutrophils. A distinctive histochemical finding is the presence of a few fine granules that react with periodic acid–Schiff reagent after pre-treatment with diastase.

ETIOLOGY AND PATHOGENESIS

The etiopathogenesis is unknown. Reticulohistiocytoses may represent an abnormal histiocytic reaction to different stimuli. In solitary forms of reticulohistiocytosis, local trauma may play a role; in diffuse forms, the association with internal malignancies and autoimmune disease suggests an immunological basis for the initiation of the reaction.

MANAGEMENT

The solitary form is surgically excised. In multicentric reticulohistiocytosis, therapy is usually not helpful. Anti-inflammatory drugs are ineffective. Systemic corticosteroids have a short-lasting favorable effect on articular lesions only. Azathioprine has proved to be of no benefit. Antimitotic agents (mainly cyclophosphamide) have been reported to induce regression of mucocutaneous lesions in only a few cases.

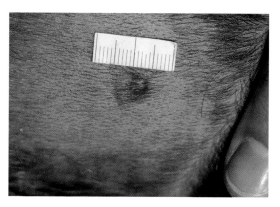

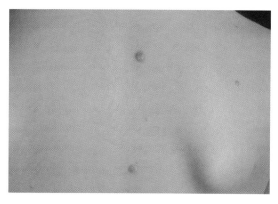

Figure 114.1

Solitary reticulohistiocytosis. An asymptomatic, dark, red, firm, dome-shaped nodule on the scalp. The patient was sent to a surgeon with the suspected diagnosis of a Spitz nevus.

Figure 114.2

Diffuse cutaneous reticulohistiocytosis. There are many papules and nodules on the trunk of this 8-year-old boy. The lesions are firm and elastic, varying in color from yellow–pink to red–brown.

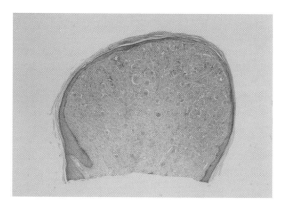

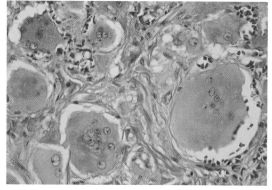

Figure 114.3

Figure 114.4

Figures 114.3 and 114.4

Reticulohistiocytosis. This nodular lesion of reticulohistiocytosis is constituted by a dense diffuse infiltrate of histiocytes with roundish nuclei and abundant granular cytoplasm. Most of the histocytes are multinucleate.

Sarcoidosis is a multisystem, granulomatous disorder of unknown cause that is uncommon in children.

EPIDEMIOLOGY

The disease occurs worldwide. Blacks are affected more often than whites. There is an equal incidence in males and females. In the majority (75% of cases) of young patients the disease appears between 8 and 15 years of age.

CLINICAL FINDINGS

Cutaneous manifestations are present in the 20–35% of patients with systemic sarcoidosis. Rarely, they are the only manifestation but more frequently they represent the first symptom. Skin sarcoidosis may manifest itself with a wide variety of skin lesions (papules, nodules or plaques). A papular rash is the commonest finding in young children and may have great diagnostic importance. It is characterized by yellow–brown, flat lesions that have a grayish–yellow color on diascopy (Figs 115.1 and 115.2). The condition begins peripherally, then becomes generalized. In children, the nodular and plaque variants are rare. These lesions consist of hard, asymptomatic, red–brown or violaceous patches, most often affecting the face and the proximal parts of the limbs.

Other types of sarcoidosis, such as angiolupoid sarcoidosis, lupus pernio, subcutaneous sarcoidosis and the erythrodermic, annular, and scar forms, are exceptional in the pediatric age group. In about 20% of adolescent females, the early stage of the disease is characterized by the appearance of an erythema nodosum. This is a non-specific manifestation, but it is considered an important favorable prognostic sign.

When the disease occurs in children under 4 years of age, it preferentially affects the skin, the joints, the eyes, and the bones, but there is no pulmonary involvement. Skin lesions usually consist of a papular rash that may precede the other symptoms by several months.

Sarcoid arthritis is the hallmark of the disease in young children, occurring in about 60% of these patients. It is persistent, non-deforming and not painful; it predominantly involves the large joints.

Eye lesions are present in about 80% of children who have arthropathy and in about 50% of patients who have generalized sarcoidosis. Uveitis is the usual and most important manifestation, and may lead to severe disability with secondary glaucoma. Conjunctivitis, retinochoroiditis, optic nerve atrophy and decreased lacrimal gland secretion may all occur.

Skeletal changes, consisting of lysis with bone cysts, have been reported in about 50% of children with sarcoidosis under the age of 4 years. These lesions are often asymptomatic and mainly involve the hands and the feet.

In patients older than 5 years of age, sarcoidosis resembles the disease in adults and principally involves the lymph nodes, the lungs and the eyes. A bilateral hilar adenopathy with pulmonary infiltrates has been demonstrated in the vast majority of older children. Dyspnea and a progressive diminution of pulmonary function are common features. Peripheral adenopathy is present in about 50% of patients. Constitutional symptoms such as weight loss, fatigue, malaise and fever are also common. Less frequently there is hepatosplenomegaly.

The course of sarcoidosis may be acute, subacute or chronic. Acute forms are characterized by erythematopapular rashes, erythema nodosum, uveitis, arthralgias and lymphadenopathy. They usually last about 2 years and tend to resolve spontaneously. Subacute and chronic forms are dermatologically characterized by nodular lesions, lupus pernio and erythrodermic manifestations, and they are associated with pulmonary, ocular and bone involvement. Their course is prolonged and progressive. The prognosis of sarcoidosis in children seems to be more favorable than in adults.

LABORATORY FINDINGS

The most common abnormal laboratory findings are hyperglobulinemia (seen in 75% of cases) and eosinophilia (in 50%). Other possible laboratory abnormalities include hypercalcemia and hypercalciuria, an elevated erythrocyte sedimentation rate, elevated alkaline phosphatase levels and neutropenia. An elevation of serum angiotensin converting factor has been observed in active phases of the disease, although patients with only skin lesions have normal levels. Many patients present cutaneous anergy, demonstrated by lack of reactivity to tuberculin and other intradermal allergens. The Kveim test yields 80–90% positive results in patients with sarcoidosis. Radiological evidence of bilateral hilar lymphadenopathy is present in about 70% of adolescents but is rare in the younger children with sarcoidosis.

HISTOPATHOLOGICAL FINDINGS

In its stereotypical presentation, sarcoidosis consists of epithelioid histiocytes arranged in collections (tubercles) that are nearly devoid of a mantle of lymphocytes or plasma cells. These tubercles, known as 'naked' tubercles, are usually present in random array throughout the dermis and rarely within the subcutaneous tissue (Figs 115.3 and 115.4). A characteristic feature of sarcoidosis is the occasional presence of fibrin in the center of some epithelioid tubercles.

ETIOLOGY AND PATHOGENESIS

The etiology of sarcoidosis remains obscure despite extensive investigations. Sarcoidosis has been considered to be a reaction pattern to various infectious agents or allergens, probably in genetically predisposed people.

MANAGEMENT

Because sarcoidosis in children is potentially self-healing, the use of systemic therapy depends on the seriousness of the internal organ involvement (i.e. ocular, lung or liver disease or hypercalcemia). Corticosteroids are the drugs of choice. The usual dosage of oral prednisone is 1 mg/kg per day for several weeks. A very gradual reduction in corticosteroid dosage is suggested in order to avoid recurrence.

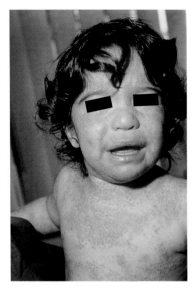

Figure 115.1
Sarcoidosis. There are numerous pink, smooth-surfaced papules, some of which tend to coalesce to form plaques.

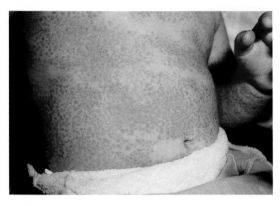

Figure 115.2
Sarcoidosis. The papules are red–brown, and some have shiny surfaces.

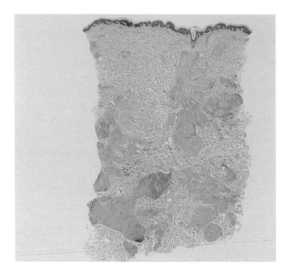

Figure 115.3

Figures 115.3 and 115.4
Sarcoidosis. Throughout the dermis are numerous, well-circumscribed, rounded or elongated aggregations of epithelioid histiocytes (tubercles), each of which is surrounded by a sprinkling of lymphocytes. Epithelioid histiocytes appear to have abundant, finely granular cytoplasm and round–oval vesicular nuclei with one or more small nucleoli.

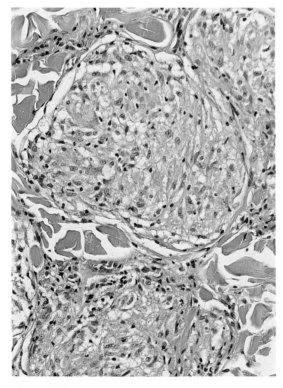

Figure 115.4

Scabies is an extremely contagious, epidemic disease that is characterized by severe itching. It is caused by the mite *Sarcoptes scabiei* var. *hominis*.

EPIDEMIOLOGY

Scabies is found universally and has epidemic outbursts that affect all races and social classes. The disease is commonest in children and young adults, but it may occur at any age.

CLINICAL FINDINGS

The pathognomonic skin lesions of scabies are burrows that appear as grayish-white, tortuous ridges several millimeters in length. The burrows are terminally capped by a small vesicle that is the resting place of the mite (Fig. 116.1). The lesions are usually found in areas with few or no hair follicles and where the stratum corneum is thin and soft. They occur most frequently in the finger webs, the volar aspects of the wrists, the axillae and, in infants, on the palms and soles. Itching is severe and intractable, particularly during the night and when the patient is warm. Secondary, non-pathognomonic lesions of scabies, caused by scratching, inappropriate treatments or hypersensitivity reactions, include papules, vesicles, pustules and excoriations that may be found all over the surface of the skin. When treatment is not undertaken early, children may have red–brown nodules (nodular scabies) that persist for a long time in spite of treatment (Fig. 116.2). Nodular lesions occur mainly on the covered parts of the body where the skin is thinnest, such as the genitalia and the axillary folds, and it is especially frequent in children aged less than 5 years.

Variants of the typical presentation of scabies include Norwegian scabies and neonatal scabies. Norwegian scabies (or crusted scabies) (Fig. 116.3) usually occurs in immunologically compromised people and is characterized by hyperkeratotic and crusted lesions of the palms and soles; these lesions are rich in parasites. This form may also involve the trunk, face, and scalp. The nails may be involved and appear dystrophic. Pruritus is mild and often absent. Neonatal scabies closely resembles Norwegian scabies and is characterized by a widespread eruption of vesicles, pustules and crusts involving all body areas, including the face. The neonates are not immunocompromised, and pruritus is absent. If not treated, the disease becomes chronic, and lichenification and nodular lesions occur. Pruritus often persists up to several weeks after eradication of mite infestation, an expression of a hypersensitivity phenomenon to mite antigens.

Complications

In infants and young children, secondary infections, such as staphylococcal and streptococcal impetigo, and eczematization are common. Streptococcal infections may give rise to acute glomerulonephritis.

LABORATORY FINDINGS

The diagnosis must be confirmed from a skin scraping of a burrow. Three findings are diagnostic – mites, their eggs and their fecal pellets. In infants, eosinophilia is frequently seen.

Histopathological findings

The papular or nodular lesions of scabies are characterized by a superficial and deep, perivascular and interstitial, mixed cell infiltrate composed almost entirely of lymphocytes and eosinophils.

Papulovesicular lesions of scabies are marked by focal spongiosis and, at times, by spongiotic vesicles. In both papules and papulovesicles of scabies, the female mite, her ova and her progeny, in the form of nymphs and larvae, may be seen within tunnels (burrows) in the cornified layer (Fig. 116.4). Fecal nuggets may also be housed within the burrow.

Norwegian scabies, also known as hyperkeratotic crusted scabies, is typified by extreme orthokeratosis and parakeratosis, throughout which mites at all stages of evolution can be observed in quantity. The cornified layer of Norwegian scabies is peppered by ova, larvae, nymphs and adult mites, as well as by numerous egg shells and countless fecal nuggets.

Etiology and pathogenesis

Scabies is caused by the female of *Sarcoptes scabiei* var. *hominis*. The mite burrows deeply into the stratum corneum and deposits her eggs. She favors areas where the stratum corneum is thin, and this fact may explain the different distribution of the lesion in children and adults. Nodular lesions seem to be due to allergic sensitivity to the mite and its products. Transmission occurs especially from close personal contact (e.g. from mothers or baby-sitters to children). The incubation period is variable; pruritus usually begins within 1 month after exposure.

Management

After a cleaning bath, different scabicides may be applied (e.g. gamma-benzene hexachloride, mesulfene, benzylbenzoate, crotamiton, permethrin). Prolonged treatments should be avoided to prevent irritation and toxicity. Permethrin is recommended in scabies therapy in premature infants, small children, patients with neurological complications and nursing mothers. All members of a family or even an entire community should undergo treatment. Cloths and bedsheets should be sterilized. In nodular scabies, preparations of coal tars should be used.

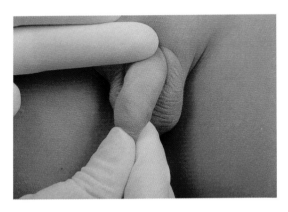

Figure 116.1
Scabies. Burrows are easily found in areas where the stratum corneum is thin and soft.

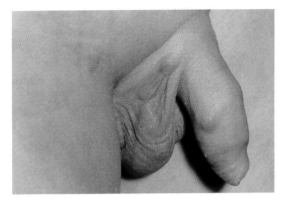

Figure 116.2
Scabies. These inflammatory, intensely itching nodules represent a variable diagnostic clue if burrows are absent or difficult to find.

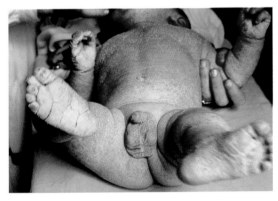

Figure 116.3
Norwegian scabies. In addition to widespread, reddish papules, some of which are scaly and which have become confluent; massive hyperkeratosis is also present on the sole.

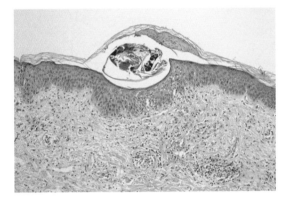

Figure 116.4
Scabies. This papular lesion of scabies shows a superficial and mid-dermal, perivascular and interstitial dermatitis constituted mostly of lymphocytes and eosinophils. The epidermis is slightly spongiotic, and the female scabies mite is housed in burrows within the cornified layer.

Scleroderma describes a group of diseases characterized by dermal hardening. These disorders range from solely cutaneous (morphea) to systemic forms (progressive systemic scleroderma).

MORPHEA

The solely cutaneous form affects all races. Females are three times as frequently affected as males. In 10–25% of cases the disease has its onset in childhood.

CLINICAL FINDINGS

Morphea includes several clinical subsets.

Plaque morphea is the most frequent type of localized scleroderma, accounting for approximately 70% of pediatric cases. It especially involves the trunk. Typically, lesions are oval in shape with a diameter of a few centimeters. The lesions are characterized by circumscribed, indurated, alopecic, ivory-colored patches (Fig. 117.1). The disease may consist of a single lesion or several asymmetrically distributed lesions. In active disease, the lesions may be prickly or slightly painful and are surrounded by a violaceous rim (lilac ring). Within the sclerodermic patches, telangiectasias can be occasionally seen and vesicobullous lesions may develop. Plaque morphea tends to show a spontaneous resolution in a few years. Healed lesions leave hyperpigmented, brownish patches that are not indurated.

Guttate morphea appears as multiple, round or oval, chalky-white lesions a few millimeters in diameter. They are characterized by minimal sclerosis and involve the shoulders, the neck and the chest. The lesions tend to remain stable.

Morphea profunda is a newly recognized subtype of localized scleroderma. It is characterized by multiple, non-tender, deep indurations. The lesions are localized in the deep dermis, the subcutaneous plane and the fascia. The overlying skin is usually brown in color. Typical patches of plaque morphea may coexist. The course is chronic and persistent.

Linear morphea accounts for approximately 18% of cases of localized scleroderma in pediatric patients. In about 20% of cases, one or more triggering factors, such as fever or trauma, can be identified. Linear morphea occurs as a hypopigmented, sclerotic, band-like lesion arising mainly on the lower extremities (Fig. 117.2). Less commonly it affects the anterior scalp, the frontal region of the head (Fig. 117.3), the arms and the anterior thorax. The disease tends to worsen and to involve the underlying tissues, and it therefore may produce severe deformities as a result of ankyloses and muscular contractures. These phenomena are especially common in children and result in impaired growth of the affected extremity. Patients with linear morphea may develop systemic autoimmune diseases.

Romberg's hemiatrophy is a segmental morphea that affects one side of the face (Fig. 117.4). As in linear morphea, the process affects not only the skin and subcutaneous fat, but also fascia, skeletal muscles and bones. Sometimes a linear morphea of the anterior scalp may coexist.

Generalized morphea is characterized by wide, hyperpigmented, sclerotic lesions diffusely involving the skin of the trunk and the thighs, while acral areas are usually spared. The disease spreads centrifugally. Sometimes the underlying muscles may be affected. Visceral involvement is rare. The disease tends to show improvement, but it persists for many years.

Disabling pansclerotic morphea of children is a recently recognized, severe variety of morphea, in which several types of localized scleroderma are combined. It accounts for approximately 2% of morphea varieties in childhood. The disease may start from a linear morphea. In this latter form, the lesions also involve subcutis, fascia, muscles and bones (Fig. 117.5). Extensor and acral areas are most commonly affected, with sparing of the fingertips and the toes, but the disease may affect also the scalp and the face. Arthralgia and severe pain caused by involvement of nerves may occur. Despite widespread and severe cutaneous involvement, Raynaud's phenomenon and signs of systemic scleroderma are usually absent. The course is progressive.

Eosinophilic fasciitis usually affects the distal area of a limb. It usually starts after physical exertion and is characterized by an area of tenderness and swelling with a cobblestone aspect on the overlying skin. The affected area subsequently becomes indurated. The disease usually regresses spontaneously or after corticosteroid treatment.

Pasini–Pierini atrophoderma usually appears on the trunk and is characterized by multiple atrophic lesions with a typical 'cliff-drop' border. The lesions are oval in shape with sizes ranging from a few millimeters to some centimeters in diameter. Concomitant lesions of typical plaque morphea have been described. The lesions are permanent.

LABORATORY FINDINGS

Eosinophilia has been reported in 30% of patients with localized scleroderma and in 80% of those with eosinophilic fasciitis. It is more common in linear morphea and in generalized morphea than in plaque morphea, and it seems to be related to the activity of the disease. Several serological findings typical of systemic autoimmune disorders have been reported. These include positivity for anti-nuclear antibodies, anti-ssDNA, anti-dsDNA, anti-centromere antibodies, anti-SCL 70 antibodies, and rheumatoid factors. These autoantibodies have been found in 31–57% of pediatric patients, with the highest percentage in linear morphea. Among children affected by linear morphea, the presence of ssDNA antibodies seems to define a subgroup with more severe and more extensive tissue involvement.

PROGRESSIVE SYSTEMIC SCLERODERMA

Progressive systemic scleroderma is a multisystemic disease with wide variations in its clinical appearance. It is very rare in children. Females are affected at a rate five times higher than males. In less than 2% of patients is the onset under 9 years of age. Two major subtypes can be identified according to the cutaneous involvement – acroscleroderma and diffuse cutaneous systemic scleroderma.

In acroscleroderma, the skin involvement starts from the fingers, the hands and the face. Raynaud's phenomenon is usually present and may precede the skin lesions by years. In the early phases of the disease, the skin of the hands is slightly swollen, owing to a non-pitting edema, and this causes reduced mobility of the fingers. A new, recently described cutaneous marker of early acroscleroderma is represented by the 'round fingerpad' sign. This consists of the disappearance of the usual contour on fingerpads, which is replaced by a hemispheric contour. Gradually, skin hardening and sclerosis with hair loss and anhidrosis develop. Later, skin atrophy and telangiectases are evident and subsequently areas of calcinosis and painful ulcers on the fingertips may develop (Fig. 117.6). Ungual lesions consist of pronounced nail fold hyperkeratosis, spots of nail fold bleeding, and telangiectasia of nail fold capillaries. A particular variant of acroscleroderma is the 'CREST' syndrome (extensive Calcinosis cutis, Raynaud's phenomenon, dysphagia caused by Esophageal involvement, Sclerodactyly and widespread Telangiectasias). This variety of progressive systemic sclerosis is seen mainly in adults.

Diffuse cutaneous systemic scleroderma accounts for only 5% of cases of progressive systemic sclerosis. It usually starts from the trunk, sparing the acral portion of the body. Raynaud's phenomenon is usually absent. Sclerosis soon involves the whole integument.

From these two extreme grades of cutaneous involvement, transitional forms of progressive systemic scleroderma exist in which the early acral scleroderma soon extends to proximal areas of the body.

Pigmentary abnormalities are commonly seen. They consist of:

- focal patches of hypopigmentation and hyperpigmentation within sclerotic areas;
- generalized brown hyperpigmentation that resembles the skin discoloration seen in adrenal insufficiency;
- perifollicular pigmentation within patches of complete pigment loss, which mimics a repigmenting vitiligo.

Joint involvement with arthralgias is common, and sometimes ankylosis may develop. Multivisceral involvement is frequent.

To summarize – the gastrointestinal tract is frequently involved in childhood progressive systemic scleroderma, and dysphagia is present in about 20% of cases and may cause chronic aspiration pneumonia; diverticula of the colon are common. Primary pulmonary involvement may be asymptomatic; it consists of restrictive changes and impaired diffusion capacity. Myocardial and pericardial involvement may be severe and may be heralded by chest pain, angina pectoris, dyspnea and syncope. Hypertension is suggestive of renal involvement. A wide spectrum of renal involvement may occur, ranging from chronic, slowly progressive renal disease to the life-threatening renal crisis of acute scleroderma. This is usually preceded by a rapid worsening and extension of the skin involvement and is characterized by severe hypertension, convulsions and oliguria or anuria. In childhood the clinical manifestations of progressive systemic scleroderma are frequently atypical and the clinical aspects are extremely variable; sometimes there are features that overlap with other autoimmune connective tissue disorders. The course is chronic. Patients with skin hardening confined to the hands have a milder course than patients with extensive skin involvement. The prognosis is determined by cardiac and renal involvement.

LABORATORY FINDINGS

The main laboratory findings in scleroderma are:

- antinuclear antibodies, which are detected in the serum of 80% of patients with acrosclerosis and in 95% of patients with diffuse scleroderma;
- antinucleolar antibodies, which are present in fewer patients;
- anticentromere antibodies, which occur in 20% of patients with diffuse scleroderma and in 70% with CREST syndrome;
- anti-scleroderma 70 antibodies, which are detected in about 30% of patients.

Several circulating antibodies directed against a wide variety of nuclear and nucleolar antigens have been found in the serum of more than 95% of patients. Non-specific laboratory abnormalities consist mainly of an increased erythrocyte sedimentation rate, raised gammaglobulin levels and mild normochromic normocytic anemia. Hemolytic anemia and thrombocytopenia may also be found. Renal involvement is revealed by increased blood urea nitrogen, high levels of plasma creatinine and mild proteinuria. In children, the commonest radiographic abnormalities are dermal and subcutaneous calcifications in periarticular areas of the fingers.

HISTOPATHOLOGICAL FINDINGS

The histological findings are similar in all forms of scleroderma. The early changes are characterized by perivascular and interstitial infiltrate that affects the dermis, the septa in

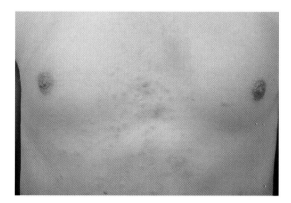

Figure 121.1
Steatocystoma multiplex. These firm asymptomatic cysts are covered by normal skin. The anterior chest is a site of predilection.

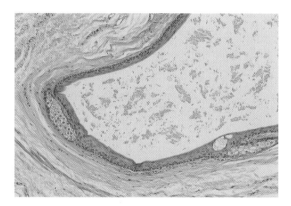

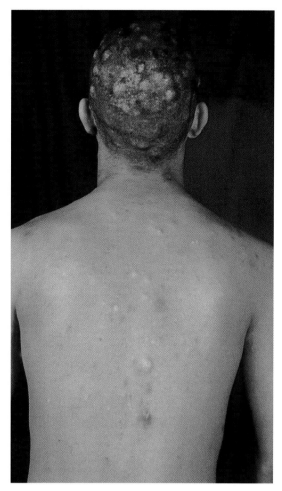

Figure 121.3
Steatocystoma. A large cystic hamartoma is situated in the dermis and subcutaneous tissue. The cyst wall is thin and is characterized by a crenulated, orthokeratotic cornified layer and the absence of the granular zone. Small sebaceous lobules connect with the cystic cavity by a sebaceous duct. Note that the cystic cavity contains sebum.

Figure 121.2
Steatocystoma multiplex. There are multiple, dome-shaped, papular lesions on the trunk that represent cysts of steatocystoma multiplex. The scalp is also extensively involved by the process.

SUBCUTANEOUS FAT NECROSIS OF THE NEWBORN

Subcutaneous fat necrosis is a rare disease affecting the panniculus of the newborn.

CLINICAL FINDINGS

Subcutaneous fat necrosis is generally noted during the 1st week of life in full-term newborns as a hardening and thickening of some areas of the skin. A careful examination reveals several painless nodules, frequently coalescent in plaques, covered by normal or erythematous skin. They are usually located on the upper part of the back (Figs 122.1 and 122.2), and the deltoids, the buttocks, the arms or the thighs, and sometimes the cheeks may be involved. The nodules are freely movable over the muscles and bones. The lesions appear rapidly but develop gradually. The indurated plaques disappear spontaneously in several weeks to months and usually without problems. Patients appear well and afebrile.

Complications

Complications occur in those cases in which nodules undergo colliquation and drain spontaneously.

HISTOPATHOLOGICAL FINDINGS

Subcutaneous fat necrosis is characterized, at scanning magnification, by a patchy infiltrate of inflammatory cells throughout lobules in the subcutaneous fat (Figs 122.3 and 122.4). At higher magnification, the infiltrate is seen to consist mostly of histiocytes, many of which possess foamy cytoplasm. Often, these foamy cells are multinucleate. Lymphocytes in variable numbers accompany the histiocytes. The crucial finding is the presence of needle-like clefts in occasional foamy histiocytes and, less commonly, in adipocytes themselves.

ETIOLOGY AND PATHOGENESIS

The etiopathogenesis is obscure. Many factors may trigger the process, including cold, trauma *in utero*, obstetrical trauma, poor nutrition, infections and biochemical defects.

MANAGEMENT

No treatment is required.

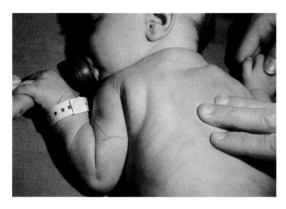

Figure 122.1
Subcutaneous fat necrosis. Numerous, non-scaly, reddish patches and plaques are a consequence of involvement by subcutaneous fat necrosis, mostly of the subcutaneous fat.

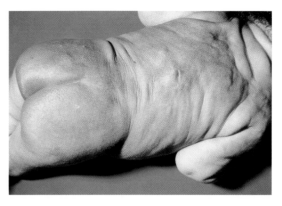

Figure 122.2
Subcutaneous fat necrosis. There is a diffuse nodularity of the skin surface, and the skin overlying the nodules is hyperpigmented.

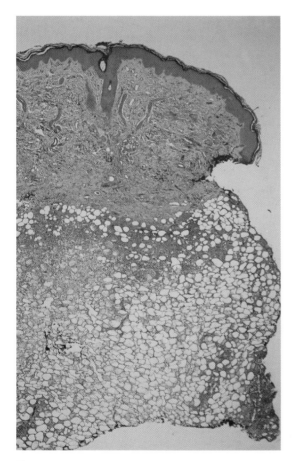

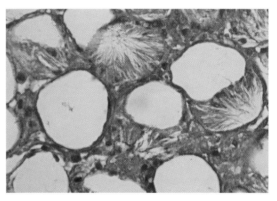

Figure 122.4

Figures 122.3 and 122.4
Subcutaneous fat necrosis. At scanning magnification, areas of necrosis and a scant inflammatory infiltrate diffusely involves fat lobules. At higher magnification (Fig. 122.4), the infiltrate consists of histiocytes, some of which contain crystals within the cytoplasm.

Figure 122.3

Sweet's syndrome (acute febrile neutrophilic dermatosis) is characterized by an explosive onset of painful, dark red macules that quickly evolve into papules and plaques, especially on the limbs, as well as fever, arthralgia and neutrophilia, all of which follow a viral syndrome.

EPIDEMIOLOGY

Sweet's syndrome is rare in childhood. The age of onset ranges between 3 months and 12 years.

CLINICAL FINDINGS

Painful dusky pink violaceous papules and nodules coalesce to form sharply demarcated plaques (Figs 123.1 and 123.2). The plaques expand centrifugally to form rings and leave postinflammatory hyperpigmentation in their centers. Advanced lesions may show tiny vesicles or pustules at their margins. There is no ulceration or scarring. Plaques tend to be asymmetrical; they may occur at any site but show a predilection for the face (see Fig. 123.1), the neck and the upper extremities (see Fig. 123.2). Patients commonly complain of high fever, malaise, headaches, arthralgias, conjunctivitis and episcleritis. On occasion, Sweet's syndrome is not accompanied by an acute onset of fever or peripheral neutrophilia. Untreated skin lesions resolve spontaneously, although resolution may take up to a few months. More than one-half of patients have recurrences, which often affect previously involved sites.

Associations

An upper respiratory infection (including tonsillitis and epiglossitis) and high fever precede the skin lesions by several days. Between 10 and 15% of adults with Sweet's syndrome have malignant neoplastic diseases, most commonly acute myelogenous leukemia.

LABORATORY FINDINGS

Peripheral leukocytosis with neutrophilia (15,000–25,000/mm³ with 90% neutrophils) is a common feature, but peripheral eosinophilia (greater than 500/mm³) and thrombocytosis (occasionally exceeding 10/mm³) may be seen. An elevated erythrocyte sedimentation rate is the most consistent laboratory abnormality.

HISTOPATHOLOGICAL FINDINGS

The most striking findings are a dense, nodular or diffuse, predominantly neutrophilic infiltrate within the reticular dermis and marked edema of the papillary dermis (Figs 123.3 and 123.4). The infiltrate, which may also contain eosinophils and be associated with extravasated erythrocytes, first presents in the upper half of the dermis and then extends throughout the dermis. Although there may be abundant nuclear 'dust', no fibrin is present in the walls of venules, an indication that there is no vasculitis. The papillary dermis often is so markedly edematous that subepidermal vesiculation seems incipient.

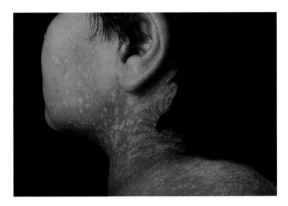

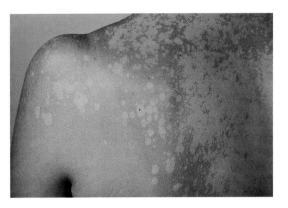

Figure 128.1

Tinea versicolor. Hypopigmented patches extend to the face, which is rarely affected in adults. Many of the spores and hyphae of *M. furfur*, the causative organism of tinea versicolor, are present in the cornified layers of the hypopigmented zones.

Figure 128.2

Tinea versicolor. There are numerous, hypopigmented macules and patches that tend to coalesce.

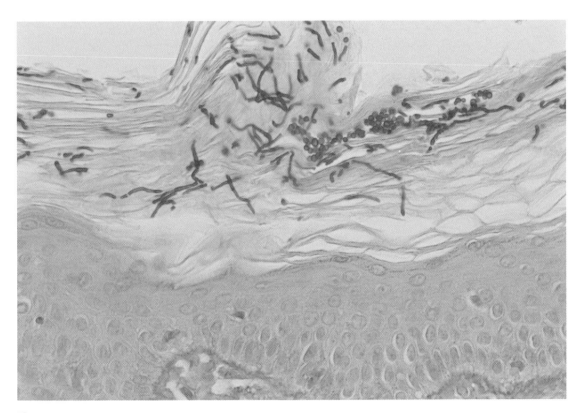

Figure 128.3

Tinea versicolor. At scanning magnification this lesion is typified by laminar hyperkeratosis and a sparse lymphocytic infiltrate around the vessels of the superficial plexus. Within the cornified layer there are short, broad hyphae and collections of round basophilic spores, a combination that has been named 'spaghetti and meatballs'. Fungal elements are better seen with periodic acid–Schiff stain.

TRICHOEPITHELIOMA

Trichoepithelioma is an uncommon, benign neoplasm of hair follicle differentiation. It affects mainly females.

CLINICAL FINDINGS

Trichoepithelioma in children occurs either as a multiple form or as a solitary form.

Multiple trichoepithelioma is characterized by numerous round, firm, pink or skin-colored, sometimes translucent nodules of 2–5 mm in diameter. The nodules are symmetrically distributed in the nasolabial folds, on the cheeks and on the eyelids (Figs 129.1 and 129.2). The number of tumors may increase over the years.

Solitary trichoepithelioma consists of a skin-colored, round, smooth, firm, asymptomatic nodule usually not more than 10 mm in diameter. The face is the most usual site.

HISTOPATHOLOGICAL FINDINGS

Trichoepitheliomas are symmetrical, well-circumscribed dermal neoplasms composed mostly of follicular germinative cells that are usually arranged in a cribriform pattern (Figs 129.3 and 129.4).

MANAGEMENT

In multiple trichoepithelioma, cryotherapy, electrodesiccation and carbon dioxide laser therapy give variable cosmetic results. In solitary trichoepithelioma, surgical excision is recommended.

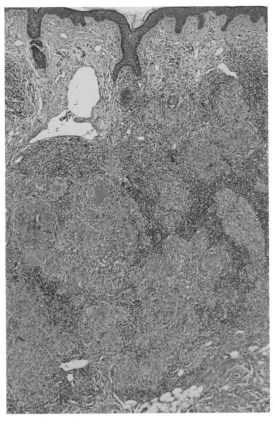

Figure 130.5

Figures 130.5 and 130.6
Lupus vulgaris. This lesion is characterized by many granulomas situated in the reticular dermis. These granulomas are constituted of collections of epithelioid cells and numerous giant cells. Note that each granuloma is surrounded by a dense infiltrate of lymphocytes. The epidermis is unaffected.

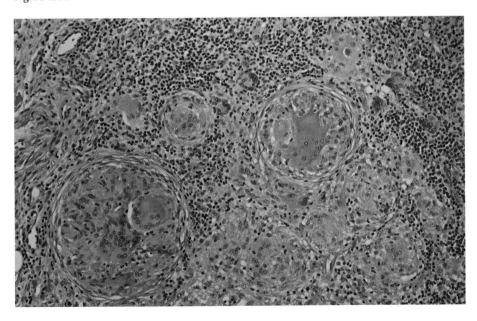

Figure 130.6

Tuberous sclerosis (epiloia, Pringle–Bourneville's disease) is a multisystemic hamartomatosis that involves the skin, the central nervous system, the eyes, the heart, the kidneys and the bones. The most characteristic features of this disorder are skin lesions, epilepsy and mental retardation.

EPIDEMIOLOGY

Tuberous sclerosis occurs in all races. Its incidence has been estimated to be 1 in 10,000.

CLINICAL FINDINGS

The skin lesions that are pathognomonic of tuberous sclerosis are angiofibromas, periungual fibromas, shagreen patches, and ash-leaf white spots. Facial angiofibromas, the so-called adenoma sebaceum of Pringle, usually become evident during childhood and are present in 80% of cases as pink–red, smooth, firm papules, 1–10 mm in diameter and symmetrically situated on the nasolabial folds, the cheeks and the chin (Fig. 131.1). Such lesions grow steadily in number and size with age. Periungual fibromas (Koenen's tumors) appear at puberty in 50% of patients as flesh-colored, elongated excrescences that emerge from the nailbed and folds (Fig. 131.2). Shagreen patches are connective tissue nevi of the collagen type; in 20–40% of cases they occur on the lumbosacral region during early childhood as yellowish orange, soft, irregular plaques, 10–100 mm in diameter (Fig. 131.3). Hypopigmented lance–ovate macules (ash-leaf spots) are found in 90% of patients at birth and represent an early diagnostic marker of this disorder. They are variable in size and number, are usually situated on the trunk (Fig. 131.4) and the limbs, and are most easily detectable by examination under Wood's light. These lesions do not alter their shapes and size with age.

Nervous system involvement occurs in about 70% of patients and consists mostly of mental retardation and epilepsy. Epilepsy usually develops during infancy or childhood, thus preceding the skin lesions.

Ocular involvement occurs in about 50% of cases and is characterized by retinal hamartomas and hamartomas of the optic nerves.

Renal involvement consists of angiolipomas (occurring in 60% of patients) and cysts (occurring in 20%).

Cardiac rhabdomyomas are associated with tuberous sclerosis in over 50% of infants. These tumors are often asymptomatic and may be self-healing. Frequently they represent, at birth, the first manifestation of the disease and are detectable by echocardiography.

Skeletal involvement, detectable in about 50% of patients using routine radiography and computed tomography, is represented by sclerotic patches, pseudocysts and periosteal new bone.

LABORATORY FINDINGS

Sclerotic calcifications in the brain are visible by computed tomography in about 50% of patients.

HISTOPATHOLOGICAL FINDINGS

Adenoma sebaceum is a hamartoma composed of fibrocytic, follicular, vascular and sometimes melanocytic elements (Figs 131.5 and 131.6).

Periungual and subungual fibromas consist of polypoid lesions in an epidermis of normal volar skin. The lesions are composed of thick bundles of collagen in vertical array in concert with an increased number of venules.

Shagreen patches are collagenous nevi marked by a papillated surface and thick bundles of collagen in the reticular dermis that are oriented perpendicular to the skin surface.

Ash-leaf spots are characterized by a normal complement of melanocytes with a decreased amount of melanin within the epidermis.

ETIOLOGY AND PATHOGENESIS

Tuberous sclerosis is inherited as an autosomal-dominant trait that shows great variability. The genes for tuberous sclerosis have been located in chromosomes 16p13 and 9q34.

MANAGEMENT

Facial angiofibromas may be treated with diathermy, dermabrasion or argon laser therapy for cosmetic reasons. Anticonvulsive drugs are moderately useful. Genetic counseling of affected patients and their families should be undertaken with care in order to identify any minimal sign of the disease in apparently unaffected parents and relatives.

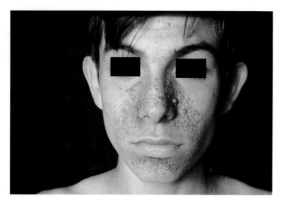

Figure 131.1
Facial angiofibromas. There are many smooth-surfaced, skin-colored and slightly brownish papules.

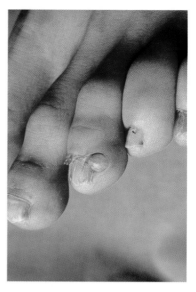

Figure 131.2
Periungual fibromas (Koenen's tumors). These somewhat warty, firm papules may be present at the sides of nail plates, as shown here, or beneath them. Because of their shape, they have also been called 'garlic clove' tumors.

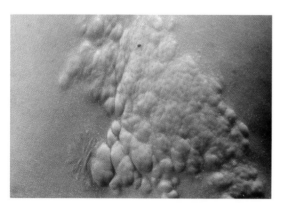

Figure 131.3
Shagreen plaque of tuberous sclerosis. This plaque, with a bumpy surface, consists of numerous, closely crowded, skin-colored papules.

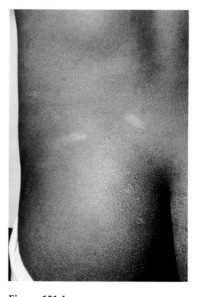

Figure 131.4
Ash-leaf spots of tuberous sclerosis. The elongated hypopigmented patches are diagnostic and are usually the first cutaneous sign of tuberous sclerosis.

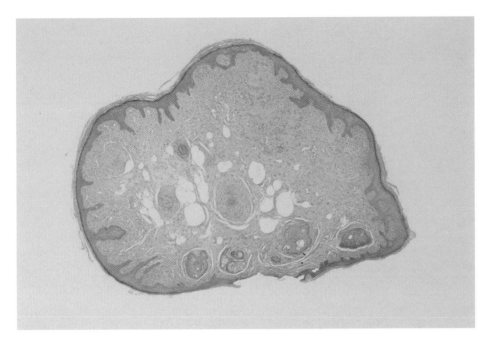

Figure 131.5

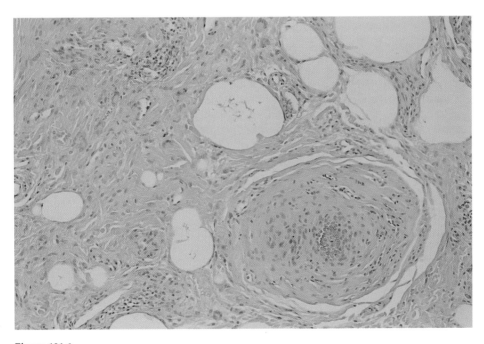

Figure 131.6

Figures 131.5 and 131.6
Adenoma sebaceum. This dome-shaped papule, which comes from a patient with tuberous sclerosis, is characterized by numerous dilated vessels, an increased number of oval and multinucleate fibrocytes, and thickened collagen bundles that are arranged in lamellae around vellus follicles.

URTICARIA AND ANGIOEDEMA

Urticaria (also known as hives or nettle rash) is any rash that is characterized by the appearance of transient elevated patches (wheals). The wheals may be redder or paler than the surrounding skin and are often itchy. In angioedema (angioneurotic edema, Quinke's edema), the lesions are deeper and may affect mucous membranes and viscera. The lesions are only mildly pruritic, if at all. Urticaria and angioedema may coexist.

EPIDEMIOLOGY

Urticaria is relatively common in children but angioedema is less so. About 10% of the general population may have had urticaria or angioedema during childhood.

CLINICAL FINDINGS

Urticaria usually presents as elevated, edematous papules of variable dimensions and redness. The shape of the lesions may be round–oval, annular, arciform or polycyclic (Fig. 132.1); their disposition is, as a rule, irregular or bizarre, except for special forms of urticaria (e.g. light urticaria, dermographism). The erythema may vary from case to case, but when the edema of the lesions is intense, it provokes a pallor in the central area of the wheal. The characteristic hard elastic consistency of the wheal may be felt easily only in large, well-elevated lesions. The number of lesions may change greatly, not only from patient to patient but also in the same patient,

depending on the degree of activity. The term 'giant urticaria' is usually used when broad, elevated patches involve the majority of the tegument. Individual urticarial lesions are relatively evanescent and last for less than 24 hours. So-called cholinergic urticaria is characterized by numerous, small wheals (2–5 mm in diameter) surrounded by an erythematous halo and usually located on the upper trunk. This form of urticaria occurs most commonly after physical or psychological stress or ingestion of spicy food or hot beverages. The course of urticaria in children is usually short (acute urticaria), but in some cases it may last for months (chronic urticaria).

When the process involves the deeper, more distensible portions of the skin, the condition is known as angioedema. In this form the depth of the edema makes the borders of the lesions, which are usually large and easily confluent (Fig. 132.2), less defined. Angioedema may be accompanied by systemic symptoms, such as fever, arthralgias, abdominal pain, vomiting, diarrhea, headache, dizziness and shock. To date it has not proved possible to suspect the cause of urticaria from the clinical appearance of the lesions.

Complications

There are no major complications from urticaria that is confined to the skin. More serious is the involvement of vital structures by angioedema. When angioedema involves the tongue and the larynx, respiratory compromise may be sufficiently severe to cause death.

HISTOPATHOLOGICAL FINDINGS

Fully developed lesions of urticaria are typified by sparse, superficial, and often superficial and deep, perivascular and interstitial infiltrates composed mostly of neutrophils and eosinophils (Figs 132.3 and 132.4). The epidermis is entirely unaffected, as is the dermoepidermal junction. Edema in urticaria forms mostly in the reticular dermis.

ETIOLOGY AND PATHOGENESIS

Although urticarial lesions can be provoked by either immune or non-immune mechanisms, urticaria is usually allergic in cause, as is angioedema. Type I hypersensitivity reactions (immunoglobulin E or immunoglobulin G_4 reagin-mediated immunity) and type III hypersensitivity reactions (immune-complex reaction) are both involved in allergic urticaria. Allergens that can be identified include inhalants, ingestants, injectants, infections or infestations, and contactants. In addition to immune-mediated urticaria, there are non-allergic forms provoked by many substances. via direct liberation of vasoactive substances. Physical urticarias, such as those that are consequences of pressure, heat, cold, ultraviolet light, and cholinergic and adrenergic stimuli, also need to be considered. Hereditary angioedema results from a deficiency of C1 esterase inhibitor.

MANAGEMENT

Management of urticaria must be tailored to the cause of the urticaria, trying to eliminate the triggering factors. Allergic urticaria may be managed by antihistamines and by systemic corticosteroids. Systemic anti-H_1 antihistamines are the drugs of choice in all the forms of non-severe urticaria to control itching. The use of anti-H_2 antihistamines, such as cimetidine, which could be considered useful for a better control of the disease, is sometimes frustrating, probably because histamine is able to act, via H_2 receptors, on mast cells and basophils to stop their degranulation. The blockage of H_2 receptors would inhibit the feedback that self-regulates the histamine liberation. Among systemic anti-H_1 antihistamines, the authors prefer to use, in children, hydroxizine, ciproeptadine, or chlorpheniramine by mouth. In chronic forms, more recent, non-sedating antihistamines (e.g. terfenadine, astemizole, cetirizine, loratadine) can also be considered.

Systemic corticosteroids should be given only in severe forms that are unresponsive to antihistamines. They should be used for a limited period to avoid side effects, some of which (e.g. growth arrest) can be particularly critical in childhood.

Hereditary angioedema may be treated with danazol, which induces increased production of C1 esterase inhibitors.

Systemic corticosteroids should be administered during the flare-ups of the disease, while severe episodes must be treated in hospital with subcutaneous administration of 0.1–0.5 ml of adrenaline (epinephrine) (1:1000), forced ventilation and, if necessary, tracheostomy.

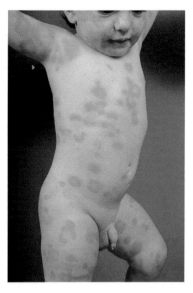

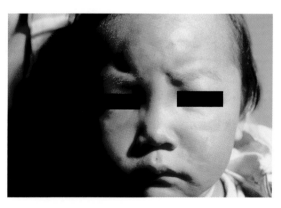

Figure 132.2
Angioedema. The eyelids, the forehead and the cheeks are markedly swollen as a consequence of edema. It is an exaggeration of urticaria at skin sites that are highly distensible.

Figure 132.1
Urticaria. The arciform or figurate arrangement of the wheals is a very characteristic pattern in infants and children.

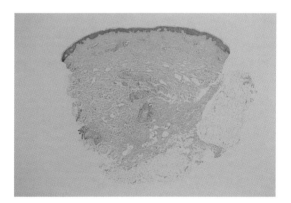

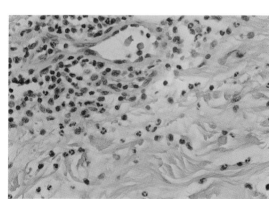

Figure 132.3   **Figure 133.4**

Figures 132.3 and 132.4
Urticaria. The specimen from which these sections were cut was taken from a child with papular and plaque lesions of urticaria. Note the superficial and deep perivascular and interstitial infiltrate composed of lymphocytes, neutrophils and some eosinophils. The epidermis is completely unaffected by the pathological process.

VARICELLA AND ZOSTER

Varicella (chickenpox) and zoster (shingles) are common, acute infectious diseases. Although they are two distinct clinical entities they are caused by the same virus. Varicella is the primary infection; zoster is a recurrence of varicella after a variable period of time and in a limited area.

EPIDEMIOLOGY

Varicella has a worldwide distribution. About 3 million cases are reported in the USA each year. The disease can develop at any age. The peak of incidence occurs from 5–9 years of age. Herpes zoster is unusual in children and exceptional in neonates.

CLINICAL FINDINGS

After a short prodromal period characterized by low fever and malaise, the disease is heralded by the appearance of a macular, pruritic rash. The lesions rapidly progress, over a few days, from macules to papules, and then to the typical 'tear-drop' vesicles on an erythematous base (Fig. 133.1). In 2–3 days the vesicles turn into pustules and the drying process begins in the center, producing an umbilicated appearance and then a crust. Lesions occur in successive crops, so that the various stages of the rash can be observed concomitantly. Characteristically the eruption is concentrated on the trunk and the head, whereas the lesions are distributed more sparsely on the face and the extremities (Fig. 133.2). Lesions also develop on the mucous membranes, especially on the palate. Itching is almost a constant feature, although it can be very variable. Healing is complete in 2–3 weeks, usually with minimal scarring. Varicella is one of the most highly communicable diseases. The average period of incubation is 15 days, and epidemics are frequent in pre-school children communities. The infectiveness of the disease is higher in the first stage of the symptoms.

Zoster in children has the same clinical features as in adults. The typical erythematovesicular rash is unilateral and limited to an area of the skin innervated by the affected sensory nerve, but usually there is no or little neuralgia. Also, fever and local lymphadenopathy are rarely encountered in children. The favorite affected area is controversial – rare on the head (Fig. 133.3), herpes zoster has a predilection for cervical (Fig. 133.4) and lumbosacral localizations, but some experts claim a high frequency on the trunk. Recovery is rapid and without sequelae in 1–2 weeks.

Complications

The most common complication of varicella is secondary bacterial infection that causes scarring of the skin. Post-zoster neuralgia is a rare occurrence in children.

LABORATORY FINDINGS

The detection of the virus can be easily obtained by Tzank's smear, which shows the typical alteration of the epithelial cells affected by the herpesvirus.

HISTOPATHOLOGICAL FINDINGS

Cutaneous infection by herpesvirus, either varicella–zoster virus or herpes simplex virus, produces predictable changes within the epidermis and epithelial structures of the adnexae – ballooned keratinocytes marked by abundant pale cytoplasm, steel–gray nuclei with margination of nucleoplasm, and the tendency to multinucleation of keratinocytes (Figs 133.5 and 133.6).

ETIOLOGY AND PATHOGENESIS

Varicella and zoster are distinct clinical entities caused by the same virus, the varicella–zoster virus.

MANAGEMENT

In normal children the treatment of both diseases is merely symptomatic with wet dressings and oral antihistamines to relieve the pruritus. Secondary bacterial infections must be prevented. In immunosuppressed patients, administration of acyclovir is useful.

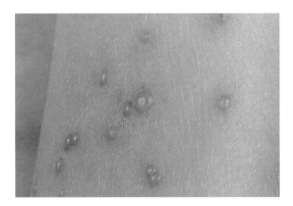

Figure 133.1
Varicella. A close view of the typical 'tear-drop' vesicles. Some of these tense vesicles, situated on slightly reddish bases, have hints of umbilication in their centers.

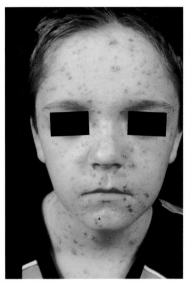

Figure 133.2
Varicella. An adolescent with a severe form of varicella. The different stages of the lesions (vesicles, pustules and crusts) are clearly visible.

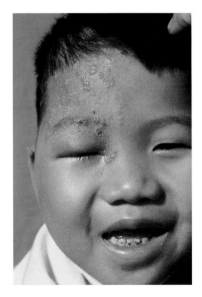

Figure 133.3
Zoster. Many tense vesicles sit on top of a broad reddish base, and the vesicles follow a dermatomal distribution limited to one side of the face. Note the marked periorbital swelling.

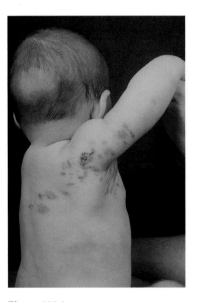

Figure 133.4
Zoster. Many vesicles and hemorrhagic crusts can be seen on an erythematous base in an infant. The lesions are distributed in a linear pattern.

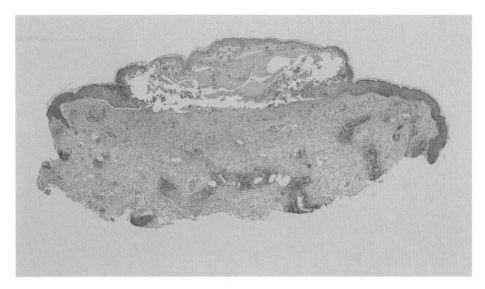

Figure 133.5

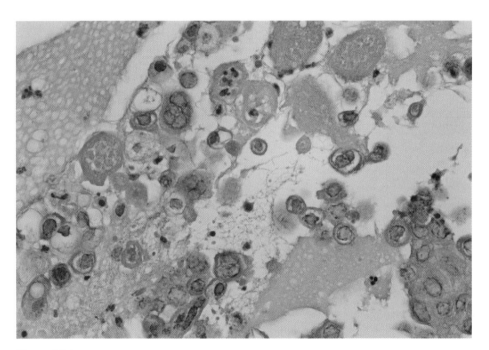

Figure 133.6

Figures 133.5 and 133.6
Herpes zoster. An intraepidermal acantholytic vesicle has become subepidermal because of the rupture of the bottom of the blister. Within the vesicle, numerous acantholytic keratinocytes with characteristic steel–gray nuclei and accentuation of the peripheral nucleoplasm, multinucleate cells and necrotic keratinocytes can be seen at higher magnification.

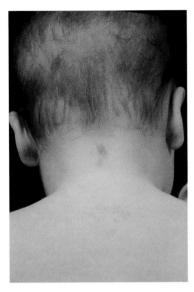

Figure 134.1
Salmon patch. This flat, rose-red irregular geographical area is localized at the nape of the neck and can be considered a normal occurrence in a Caucasian newborn.

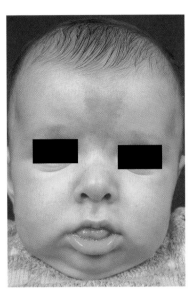

Figure 134.2
Salmon patch. This flat, rose, V-shaped patch located on the forehead can be considered normal in a Caucasian newborn. It will fade with age.

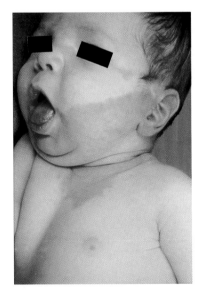

Figure 134.3
Port-wine stain. This lesion, localized unilaterally on the third branch of the trigeminal nerve, is pink–red but, unless treated, it will turn red–purple with time.

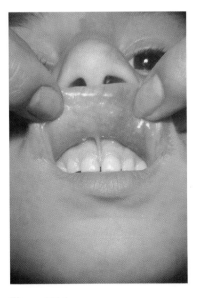

Figure 134.4
Port-wine stain. This vascular patch affects the second branch of the trigeminal nerve and not only involves the skin but also the mucosal surface.

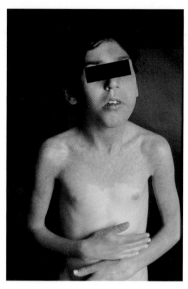

Figure 134.5
Sturge–Weber syndrome. Glaucoma and seizures are the consequences of meningeal and retinal angiomatosis in this child affected by a large capillary malformation.

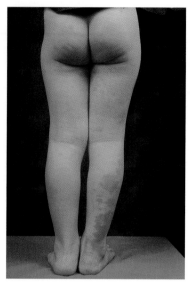

Figure 134.6
Klippel–Trenaunay syndrome. In this young girl the symmetrical involvement of the lower limbs is evident, this is due to venous malformation in association with the capillary patch of the leg.

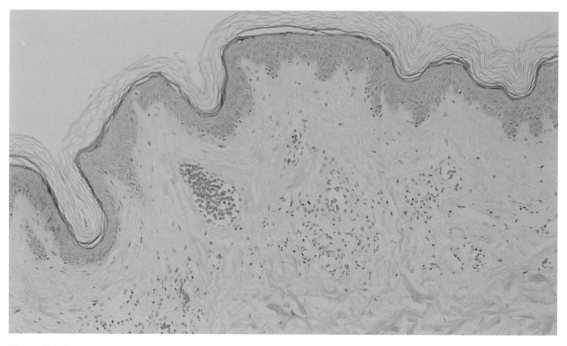

Figure 134.7
Port-wine stains. A dilation of capillaries and small venules in the superficial dermis not accompanied by endothelial cell proliferation is the histological hallmark of this malformation.

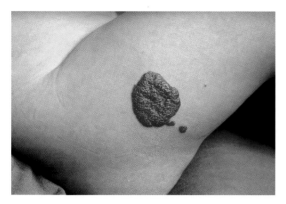

Figure 134.8
Capillary hemangioma. This well-defined vascular tumor, which has a vivid red color and a hard elastic consistency, was not present at birth. It is a superficial capillary hemangioma.

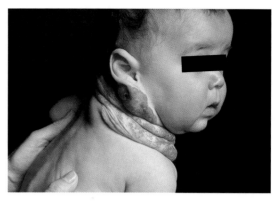

Figure 134.9
Capillary hemangioma. Huge lesions may regress but the texture of the skin is permanently altered; plastic surgery should be advised.

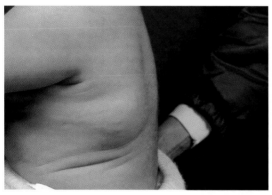

Figure 134.10
Capillary hemangioma. This round, elastic, poorly defined nodule is covered by normal skin, which has a tendency to a blue hue. Echo Doppler reveals a clear pattern of vascularization.

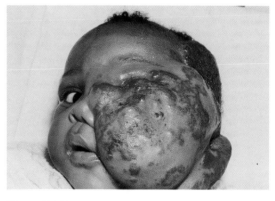

Figure 134.11
Capillary hemangioma. In this patient, this disfiguring mass is dangerous because of the risk of ulceration and visual impairment.

Figure 134.12
Capillary hemangioma. In this fully developed lesion, the vascular lumens are wide and lined by a single layer of plump endothelial cells; most of them are filled with erythrocytes.

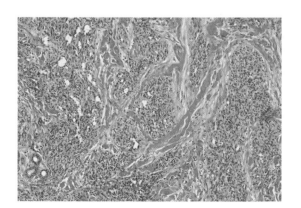

135　VITILIGO

Vitiligo is a common, acquired, circumscribed loss of cutaneous pigment caused by destruction of melanocytes.

EPIDEMIOLOGY

Vitiligo affects all races and both sexes equally and occurs in about 1% of the world's population. The mean age of onset in children has been found to range from 4.6 to 4.8 years.

CLINICAL FINDINGS

Vitiligo is characterized by chalk-white, sharply outlined patches (Fig 135.1 and 135.2) that are often surrounded by hyperpigmented borders. In the early stages the pigment loss may be partial, with various stages of light brown coloration (trichrome vitiligo). The sizes, shapes and number of lesions are very variable, but initial lesions are almost always round or oval and tend to grow centrifugally with typical convex margins. It is possible to distinguish a localized form, which involves one region of the skin, sometimes with a unilateral dermatomal array (segmental vitiligo) (see Fig. 135.2) and a generalized form, which often has a symmetrical distribution (see Fig. 135.1). Sites of predilection are the face, particularly around the eyes and the mouth, the dorsum of the hands, the axillae, the groin and the genitalia. Involvement of the palms and soles is common but evident only by Wood's lamp examination. A halo of depigmentation around a pigmented nevus (vitiligo perinevica) may be the initial symptom of the disease. Leukotrichia is relatively common in these patients and their relatives. Mucosae may also be involved, especially the genitalia, the nipples, the lips and the gingivae. The course of vitiligo is unpredictable. The disease may remain stationary, extend or progress rapidly. Spontaneous repigmentation may occur; however, such repigmentation is almost never homogeneous and presents a perifollicular distribution.

Associations

Vitiligo may be associated with other skin disorders (e.g. alopecia areata, morphea, lichen sclerosus et atrophicus, psoriasis, melanoma). Several extracutaneous conditions, mostly characterized by an autoimmune pathogenesis, may be observed in patients with vitiligo.

HISTOPATHOLOGICAL FINDINGS

Early lesions of vitiligo show a sparse superficial perivascular infiltrate of lymphocytes associated with a normal complement of melanocytes at the dermoepidermal junction and normal amounts of melanin within the epidermis. Fully developed lesions have no melanocytes and no melanin within the epidermis (Fig. 135.3).

ETIOLOGY AND PATHOGENESIS

The etiopathogenesis of vitiligo is unknown. About 30–40% of patients have a positive family history of the condition. Three major theories have been put forward to explain the cause of the disease – the autodestructive theory, the neurogenic theory, and the autoimmune theory. The autoimmune theory, the most favored, is based on the frequent association of vitiligo with other autoimmune diseases and the detection of 'vitiligo antibodies' to normal human melanocytes.

MANAGEMENT

Treatment of vitiligo is frequently unsatisfactory. Patients older than 12 years of age are generally treated with oral psoralen compounds or khellin followed by gradual exposure to sunlight or psoralen and ultraviolet-A therapy. For localized lesions in children, a topical treatment (psoralen lotion at very low concentrations) followed by short, well-controlled ultraviolet-B or ultraviolet-A exposure twice a week may be useful. Hydrocortisone has been used for repigmenting isolated small macules. Sunscreen may be useful for avoiding sunburn.

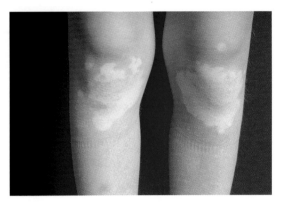

Figure 135.1
Vitiligo. Symmetrical, achromic lesions are present on the knees. A Koebner phenomenon may occur at this site after trauma.

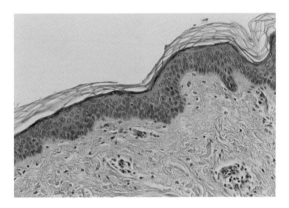

Figure 135.3
Vitiligo. In sections stained by hematoxylin and eosin, fully developed lesions of vitiligo are characterized by complete absence of melanocytes and melanin within the epidermis. A sparse perivascular lymphocytic infiltrate is present around the vessels of the superficial plexus.

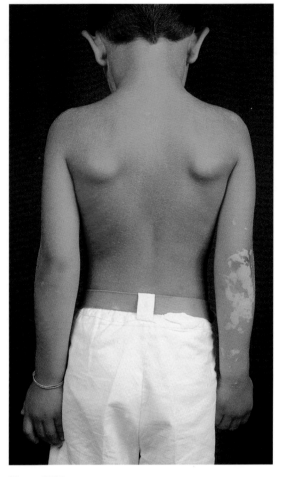

Figure 135.2
Vitiligo. The localized variant is characterized by achromic patches that involve one region of the skin, sometimes with a dermatomal distribution (segmental vitiligo).

Warts are proliferative, chronic, benign lesions of the skin and adjacent mucous membranes that are caused by epidermotropic DNA viruses of the papova goup (human papillomaviruses). Each particular type of wart has been found to be associated with an individual papillomavirus or group of papillomaviruses.

EPIDEMIOLOGY

Warts are one of the commonest dermatological disorders throughout the world. In children, warts represent 3–5% of all skin problems and generally occur during the school year.

CLINICAL FINDINGS

Common warts are typically exophytic (ie elevated) neoplasms. Their surface is hyperkeratotic and rough because of minute papillary projections, and their size varies from a few millimeters to few centimeters (Fig. 136.1). Not infrequently they are confluent and hypertrophic, especially in periungual locations. They are gray, brownish or flesh-colored, and early warts may have a smooth surface. Common warts are localized mainly on the dorsum of the hands, but they can also be palmar or plantar or can appear elsewhere on the skin, on the semimucosa (e.g. on the red of the lips), or very rarely, on mucous membranes.

Plane warts are slightly raised above the skin level, are smaller than common warts and have flatter, smoother surfaces (Fig. 136.2). More frequently they are multiple, irregularly disseminated or grouped and confluent; they are sometimes distributed in lines because of the Koebner phenomenon. They are mainly localized on the face, especially the forehead, and less commonly on the forearms.

Filiform warts are elongated and digitated excrescences that usually occur on the eyelids and around the lips and the nose (Fig. 136.3).

Plantar warts are endophytic, firm, round, painful lesions surrounded by smooth keratotic rings. They occur on the plantar surfaces of the feet. When pared they reveal small black points that represent thrombosed capillaries of dermal papillae.

Genital warts (condylomata acuminata) appear as soft, pink, elongated excrescences that tend to cornification. They occur on the genitalia and in the perianal region (Fig. 136.4). They are not common in infants and children.

Approximately two-thirds of warts resolve spontaneously within 2 years.

HISTOPATHOLOGICAL FINDINGS

Verruca vulgaris consists of papillated or digitated epidermal hyperplasia; hypergranulosis; collarettes of adnexal epithelium; and dilated, tortuous capillaries in the dermal papillae (Fig. 136.5).

Condylomata acuminata is characterized by papillated, epidermal hyperplasia; focal parakeratosis; focal hypergranulosis; and dilated, tortuous blood vessels in dermal papillae.

Verruca plana shows mammillated epidermal hyperplasia, halos around nuclei in the granular zone or vacuolated gray–blue cytoplasm in cells in the upper part of the viable epidermis; and a cornified layer marked by basket-weave configuration (Fig. 136.6)

MANAGEMENT

Wart therapy, although always challenging, presents additional dilemmas in young chidren. As in all therapeutic decisions, the risk–benefit ratio must be carefully consid-ered. Since treatment is always painful and young children usually have no desire to be treated, the situation can be traumatic for the patients, parents and doctors. One must keep in mind the great tendency for spontaneous resolution of warts and better long-term cosmetic results when that occurs. The decision regarding therapy depends on the patient's age, the type of wart, the likelihood of its spontaneous resolution, the symptoma-tology, the discomfort of the therapy, the risk of scarring and the desires of the patient's parents. A non-aggressive treatment is usually the best solution.

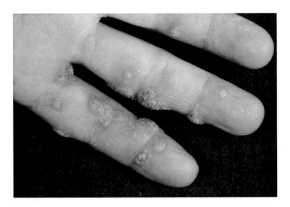

Figure 136.1
Common warts. These discrete papules are slightly papillated and hyperkeratotic.

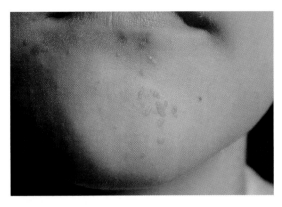

Figure 136.2
Plane warts. Numerous tan papules, some of which have become confluent, tend to be aligned in linear fashion.

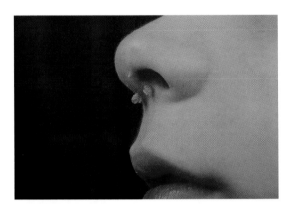

Figure 136.3
Filiform warts. Elongated and digitated excrescences on the nose.

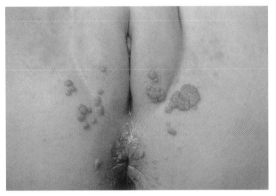

Figure 136.4
Condylomata acuminata. In this early stage in the evolution of condylomata acuminata, papules are both discrete and confluent, slightly reddish and devoid of marked hyperkeratosis. Some warty lesions are present in the perianal region.

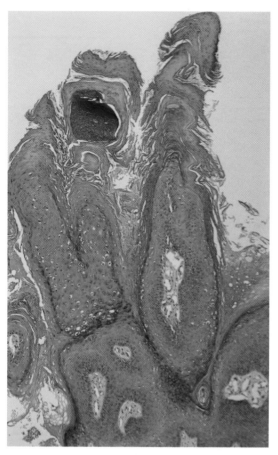

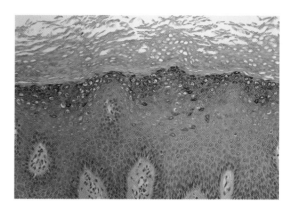

Figure 136.6
Verruca plana. Mammillated epidermal hyperplasia, orthokeratotic hyperkeratosis, hypergranulosis, and keratinocytes of the upper spinous zone and of the granular zone with blue–gray cytoplasm are characteristic histological features of plane warts.

Figure 136.5
Verruca vulgaris. A fully developed lesion of verruca vulgaris is characterized by marked digitated epidermal hyperplasia, collarettes of adnexal epithelium, prominent tortuosity of the capillaries in dermal papillae, and hypergranulosis. Parakeratosis can be seen at the tips of digitations together with collections of red cells, whereas corneocytes between these digitations are orthokeratotic. Note that keratinocytes of the granular layer have clear spaces around nuclei.

Xanthoma disseminatum or (Montgomery's syndrome) is a rare, benign, normolipemic form of histiocytoxanthomatosis. It affects the skin and mucous membranes and is frequently associated with diabetes insipidus.

EPIDEMIOLOGY

About 60% of cases of xanthoma disseminatum have their onset between the ages of 5 and 25 years.

CLINICAL FINDINGS

The cutaneous manifestations are marked by the eruption of hundreds of papules that are red–brown at first and then become yellowish. They show a predilection for the flexural surfaces and the intertriginous areas such as the axillae (Fig. 137.1), the groin, the neck, the antecubital and the popliteal fossae, the periorbital regions (Fig. 137.2) and the genitalia. The lesions, particularly those in flexures and folds, tend to merge quickly to form verrucous plaques. In about 50% of cases, xanthomatous lesions may also be observed on the mucous membranes of the mouth, the pharynx and the larynx and on the conjunctiva and the cornea. Symptoms of dyspnea and dysphagia are not uncommon. Vasopressin-sensitive transitory diabetes insipidus is present in about 40% of the cases. Polyuria and polydypsia are generally mild. Xanthoma disseminatum is essentially a self-limited disease. The skin lesions and the diabetes insipidus resolve spontaneously after several years. Only a few cases have demonstrated a progressive course.

LABORATORY FINDINGS

A normal lipid profile is a dogma of this disease.

HISTOPATHOLOGICAL FINDINGS

The papulonodular lesions are characterized by an infiltrate of large mononuclear or multinucleate foamy histiocytes intermingled with lymphocytes, plasma cells and neutrophils (Figs 137.3 and 137.4).

MANAGEMENT

Treatment is usually not helpful. Systemic corticosteroids and antimitotic agents have been used in the more disfiguring forms. Pitressin is necessary to check the diabetes insipidus.

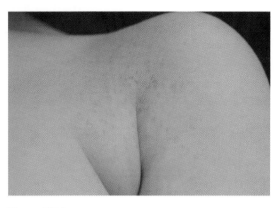

Figure 137.1
Xanthoma disseminatum. Yellow–brown papules concentrated on the axillary folds in a 5-year-old patient with diabetes insipidus.

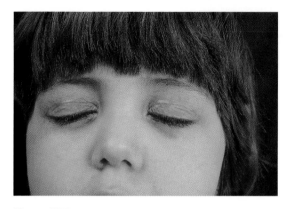

Figure 137.2
Xanthoma disseminatum. Yellow–brown papules merging into plaques are present on the eyelids of the same patient.

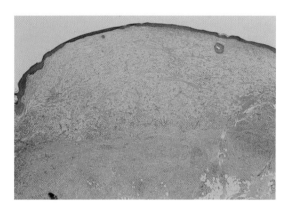

Figure 137.3

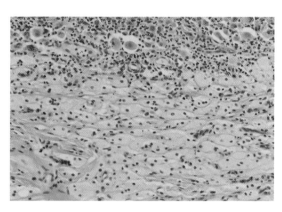

Figure 137.4

Figures 137.3 and 137.4
Xanthoma disseminatum. The majority of the cells constituting this fully developed lesion of xanthoma disseminatum are large histiocytes with vesicular nuclei and abundant foamy cytoplasm. Other cells in the infiltrate include large histiocytes with eosinophilic cytoplasm, lymphocytes, plasma cells and neutrophils.

XERODERMA PIGMENTOSUM

Xeroderma pigmentosum is a rare, hereditary disorder. It is characterized by hypersensitivity to sunlight, the early development of freckle-like lesions on photoexposed areas, skin atrophies and a high incidence of skin cancers.

EPIDEMIOLOGY

Xeroderma pigmentosum is a rare disease, occurring in about 1 in 250,000 births.

CLINICAL FINDINGS

The disease manifests itself as soon as exposure to light takes place. It is progressive, causing photophobia in newborns, the first skin changes at 1–5 years of age and skin tumors during adolescence. Neurological signs, when present, appear in early infancy. Cutaneous lesions occur predominantly, but not exclusively, on photoexposed areas, and it is possible to recognize three successive stages. At first, the skin becomes dry and erythematous, with or without blisters after sunburn. Pigmented, bizarrely shaped freckles appear and are intermingled with hypopigmented areas and telangiectasias (Fig. 138.1). In the second stage, continuous sun exposure and subsequent sunburns induce atrophy of the skin and may leave scars (e.g. mutilation of the fingertips or the ears, and ectropion). The third stage is characterized by the development of basal cell carcinomas (Fig. 138.2), squamous cell carcinomas (Fig. 138.3), keratoacanthomas, malignant melanomas and, rarely, sarcomas. The first tumors appear in childhood or adolescence and then increase in size and number. Precancerous lesions, appearing as verrucosities, cutaneous horns, bizarrely shaped lentigo maligna or even scars, arise on large areas and give the skin a characteristic reticular appearance. Ophthalmological symptoms are found in about 80% of cases and are extremely variable – photophobia and conjunctivitis are early symptoms, and corneal opacities, ulcerations, and symblepharon and ectropion occur later. Mouth lesions, such as cheilitis and freckle-like hyperpigmentation, and basal and squamous cell carcinomas of the lips may be observed. True mucous membrane lesions, such as buccal mucosa and tongue erosions and papillomas or gingivostomatitis, have been reported.

The variable degree of severity of the disease is related to the presence of different molecular defects. In the De Sanctis–Cacchione syndrome, the clinical picture of xeroderma pigmentosum is associated with neurological symptoms including microcephaly, progressive mental deterioration, low intelligence, hyporeflexia or areflexia, choreoathetosis, ataxia, spasticity and Achilles tendon shortening with eventual tetraparesis. Markedly retarded growth and hypogonadism may also occur.

LABORATORY FINDINGS

Routine laboratory tests are usually normal. Cultured cells show higher sensitivity to ultraviolet radiation-induced damage, the growth rate is reduced and the cellular recovery is delayed. There is a reduced rate of DNA synthesis. Mutations in the genes that encode for the DNA repair proteins can be detected.

HISTOPATHOLOGICAL FINDINGS

Early histological skin changes in children with xeroderma pigmentosum include evidence of premature solar elastosis, hyperkeratosis, focal atrophy of the epidermis, and a sparse lymphohistiocytic infiltrate in the papillary dermis. In some areas there is hyperpigmentation of the basal layer of the epidermis with or without an increase in the concentration of melanocytes. In time these features become more pronounced, and focally basal keratinocytes exhibit large and hyperchromatic atypical nuclei (Fig. 138.4).

ETIOLOGY AND PATHOGENESIS

Xeroderma pigmentosum is a genetically inherited disease, caused by an autosomal-recessive mutation. The clinical features result from a genetically determined defect of the enzyme system, which normally repairs the ultraviolet radiation-induced DNA damage. Complementation studies using heterokaryons have shown that at least nine complementation groups of xeroderma pigmentosum exist (from A to I), with one variant group.

MANAGEMENT

Treatment consists of life-long avoidance of exposure to the sun by using adequate protection (clothes, sunglasses and sunscreens) in order to delay the onset of the clinical symptoms and tumors. Some patients have been treated with oral retinoids for months to years in order to provide protection against tumors. Beta-carotene per os is another effective treatment in association with retinoids. In affected families, prenatal diagnosis can be performed. Precancerous lesions and skin tumors should be excised.

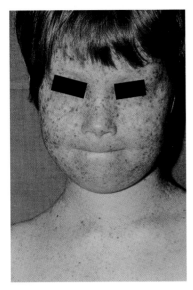

Figure 138.1
Xeroderma pigmentosum. The skin of the neck and shoulders is thin, dry and scaly with many hypopigmented and hyperpigmented macules. The combination of dyschromia, atrophy and telangiectasia is called poikiloderma.

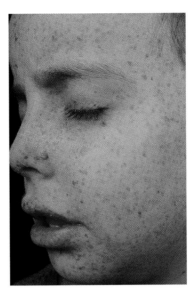

Figure 138.2
Xeroderma pigmentosum. The nodular lesion on the nose is a basal cell carcinoma.

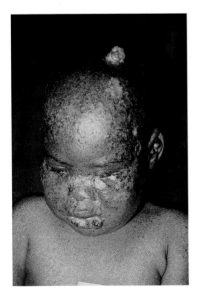

Figure 138.3
Xeroderma pigmentosum. The reticulated hypopigmentation and hyperpigmentation on the chest and the arms is typical of sun-exposed skin in xeroderma pigmentosum. On the lips, the cheeks and the forehead there are squamous cell carcinomas.

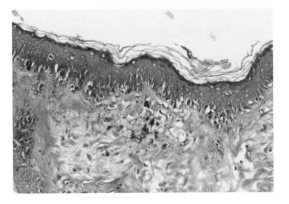

Figure 138.4
Xeroderma pigmentosum. This melanoma *in situ* developed on the face a 21-year-old patient with xeroderma pigmentosum. There are an increased number of atypical melanocytes arranged as solitary units and small nests within the epidermis. The atypical melanocytes arranged as solitary units predominate markedly over melanocytes disposed in nests. A few of the atypical melanocytes lie above the dermoepidermal junction. Note the severe solar elastosis in this section.

INDEX

Page numbers in *italics* refer to illustrations.